SUPER
M

Essential Information for Your Health and Well-Being

Discover:

- how vitamin C can minimize the intensity of hot flashes
- why drinking soda may increase your chances of developing osteoporosis
- why "healthy" polyunsaturated fats such as safflower and corn oil have been linked to a greater incidence of breast tumors
- why a fat-free diet is a dangerous diet
- how adding the right fats to your diet can reduce many of the discomforts of menopause
- why your menopausal symptoms my be related to weakened adrenal glands and how simple nutritional and lifestyle changes can dramatically lessen the severity of these symptoms
- how excess sugar consumption has been linked to calcium deficiencies and breast cancer
- why milk may be hazardous to your health—the phosphorus/calcium connection

SUPER NUTRITION
FOR
MENOPAUSE

ANN LOUISE
GITTLEMAN

POCKET BOOKS

New York   London   Toronto   Sydney   Tokyo   Singapore

The author of this book is not a physician, and the ideas, procedures, and suggestions in this book are not intended as a substitute for the medical advice of a trained health professional. All matters regarding your health require medical supervision. Consult your physician before adopting the suggestions in this book, as well as about any condition that may require diagnosis or medical attention. The author and publisher disclaim any liability arising directly or indirectly from the use of the book.

An *Original* Publication of POCKET BOOKS

POCKET BOOKS, a division of Simon & Schuster Inc.
1230 Avenue of the Americas, New York, NY 10020

ISBN: 0-671-78100-6

First Pocket Books printing October 1993

10 9 8 7 6 5 4 3

POCKET and colophon are registered trademarks of Simon & Schuster Inc.

Cover photo by Wendi Schneider

Printed in the U.S.A.

*This book is dedicated to Shira
and her generation . . . with love.*

Acknowledgments

My most sincere thanks are extended to my literary agent, Michael Cohn, who has been a wonderful friend and adviser for so many years. Thanks also to my Pocket Books editor, Denise Silvestro, whose enthusiasm and support have enabled me to create a manuscript that will hopefully reach women of all ages from all walks of life. And, of course, heartfelt thanks to my dear associate Alice Swanson, whose creative talents and "grounding" have made this book a reality. A big thank-you to John Lee, M.D., and Bruce MacFarland, Ph.D., whose research and professional reviews of my manuscript have enhanced this book.

I would also like to acknowledge my patients, whose real-life experiences have taught me so much. My appreciation is sincerely extended to natural foods cook and teacher Eleonora Manzolini for assisting in the recipe development. Last but not least, I honor two nutritional pioneers, Dr. Hazel Parcells and the late Nathan Pritikin, whose brilliance and love for humanity have been my inspiration.

Contents

Foreword

In seventeen years of holistic medical care, prescribing lifestyle modification and dietary supplements, women have accounted for well over half of my patients. However, for many years, health and medical research have rarely addressed those issues that are exclusive to women. Most studies neglected to include women in their research sample; even studies of heart disease, the number-one killer of both men and women, virtually ignored the female population.

In the past, premenstrual syndrome (PMS) and menopause have been forbidden topics. PMS was either a monthly inconvenience you had to live with or was dismissed as being "all in your head." Recent changes in attitude and the political climate have begun to lift the cloud of mystery that has enshrouded PMS. Doctors now treat PMS symptoms with numerous drugs to reduce anxiety, eliminate fluid retention, relieve headaches and manage cramps. However, little attention has been paid to how lifestyle changes and nutritional supplements can more safely control all of these symptoms. The importance of drug side effects and addictions (especially to anti-anxiety drugs) has been minimized by the medical community and the pharmaceutical industry.

The same has been true for menopause and the symptoms that may be associated with what is often called the "change of life." Menopausal symptoms were considered significant only after the medical community had developed a new understanding of the role of hormonal balance, and after they had a new drug to treat it. Although hormonal replacement therapy has its place, it has led physicians to ignore the many benefits of health-habit modification. The view of the human body as a collection of independent metabolic and hormonal functions leads to a singular approach to the management of problems. But menopause involves hormonal balance, physiology and psychology. An integrated view leads naturally to more comprehensive management.

Most people do not understand the natural changes that occur in women with the cessation of the menstrual cycle, and people fear what they do not understand. Menopause is simply another change, like puberty and childbearing. It is not something to fear, but something to prepare for and to work with.

In a sense, menopause, like milestone birthdays, is feared as a sign of aging. But the significant dangers associated with menopause, such as heart disease and osteoporosis, are really due to the accelerated aging which results from a lifetime of poor health habits (smoking, alcohol, caffeine, sedentary living, poor diet). These dangers can be minimized, or reversed, at any age by modifying lifestyle and diet, and taking nutrient supplements. Likewise, the less threatening symptoms of hot flashes, skin and vaginal dryness, depression and anxiety can be addressed without drugs or hormones.

We now know that hormonal changes both during and after the menstrual years can produce profound effects, especially when combined with inappropriate health habits and dietary imbalances and inadequacies. For a long time medicine has offered women two choices: accept the symptoms and risks as inevitable or rely on drug and hormone treatment. Now they have a healthier alternative.

For years I have counseled women to reduce the total fat, hydrogenated fat, sugar and animal products in their diets and to eliminate artificial products. I have also observed the health enhancement provided by nutritional supplements. Only recently has the use of dietary supplements been accepted beyond the treatment of deficiency diseases. We now know that vitamins, minerals and essential fatty acids can be used to treat many symptoms and diseases, to enhance immunity and longevity. They are also effective in re-establishing metabolic balance. Women have been eager to learn about and implement these changes, and they have often experienced dramatic results. This book will give many more women the same opportunity.

In *Supernutrition for Menopause,* top nutritionist Ann Louise Gittleman presents a clear analysis of the relationships between health habits and the symptoms that often accompany the period of time surrounding menopause. She demystifies the entire arena of formerly taboo subjects, and gives midlife women the opportunity to make a healthy transition to the postmenopausal years. Ann Louise makes complex problems easily understandable, and she gives specific approaches to lifestyle modifications that help to ease symptoms that may accompany hormonal and psychological changes.

Ann Louise Gittleman is well qualified to write this book. She has had many years of academic training and has maintained a private practice for twenty years. She organized the nutrition education program for Nathan Pritikin and for two years supervised the day-to-day nutrition operation at the Pritikin Longevity Center. She is currently a chairperson of the Department of Nutrition of the American Academy of Nutrition, the only accredited nutrition home-study program in the country. She is the author of the bestselling *Beyond Pritikin,* the award-winning *Supernutrition for Women,* and *Guess What Came to Dinner. Supernutrition for Menopause* is an excellent addition to her work.

Women can read this book for themselves, their mothers, daughters and granddaughters, educating many generations in life habits that will serve them well through all their years. Every transition in a woman's life can be one of pleasure and excitement in the joys of living and learning. Reading this book will help you to discover these possibilities.

Michael Janson, M.D.,
Center for Preventive Medicine

Introduction

Sometime during the next decade I, along with some 25 million other women of my baby-boom generation, will reach menopause, a major gateway in a woman's life. I wrote this book because of my experience while researching my second book, *Supernutrition for Women,* in 1988. At that time I was struck by the lack of information available on a nutritional approach to menopause, a natural event that every single female will experience. In contrast, I ran across mountains of information on diets and vitamin programs to control other female conditions such as premenstrual syndrome (PMS) and yeast, for example. The latter problems can affect up to 50 percent of women from the ages of 18 to 45, while menopause affects 100 percent of all women.

While director of nutrition at the Pritikin Longevity Center in Santa Monica, California, I saw how dramatic changes in health took place in patients with heart disease, diabetes, and hypertension once they followed a suitable diet and exercise program. After leaving Pritikin for my own practice, I worked with countless women, reviewing over 7,000 diet histories. I developed diet and supplement programs for allergies, weight loss, weight gain, eating disorders, irritable bowel syndrome, parasites, PMS, and yeast infections. Time and time again I saw how nutrition and the right supplements could prevent, control, and cure these disorders. Why not a nutrition program to prevent or control the unpleasant symptoms associated with a natural life change like menopause? Besides, as a woman now in her forties, I wanted to learn all I could about menopause, not only for my clients but for myself. You might even call this book a labor of love for enlightened self-interest.

By the time I was ready to write *Supernutrition for Menopause* in 1992, there was a flurry of menopause titles on the market. Women's magazines carried featured articles on the topic from every imaginable vantage point—social, psychological, physiological, emotional, even spiritual—but no one was talking about the nutrition connection. Menopause was virtually uncharted nutritional territory, and I felt eminently ready and qualified to take on the task of researching and developing a state-of-the-art nutrition program for the menopausal woman. Surely the information had to be out there somewhere, but no one had taken the time to put it all together or look at the situation from a nutritional point of view.

But where to begin? Like many of my contemporaries, my personal understanding was shrouded in mystery and confusion. I was completely in the dark about menopause. For centuries, most medical literature was dominated by male authors, and little was written about women and their unique problems. Nobody was talking about it at all when I was growing up in the 1950s and '60s. My mother tells me she breezed through "the change" with a minimum of hot-flash or night-sweat discomfort. She says she was so busy teaching and being involved in her women's organizations that she had no time to think about it. That was her secret. I suspect that my mother and other women who didn't experience the telltale discomforts of menopause were in good glandular health to begin with.

Professionally, I have been a nutritionist specializing in female health problems for over 15 years. My female clients in the 50-something age bracket who were approaching or had completed this midlife event never even mentioned their menopausal experiences in our counseling sessions. Generally, their diet histories indicated they watched what they ate, took vitamins, and exercised regularly, and that, as a matter of course, practically all of them took estrogen. None of them ever questioned the wisdom of taking a substance the levels of which Mother Nature saw fit to reduce in this natural transition phase of a woman's life. None of them ever sought an alternative or natural approach to estrogen replacement, so neither did I. Clearly, my own personal and professional experience had not provided the nutritional answers I was now looking for.

During my research I stumbled across an enlightening bit of information: we female humans are truly unique. Unlike the females of any other species on earth, we live beyond our years of reproduction. However, according to some researchers this is a relatively recent event in history. A century ago, the average life expectancy of a woman was only about 46 years. The average age of menopause occurrence is 51, so few women back then had the opportunity to experience it. Today life expectancy for women is 78 years. Many women will now live one-third of their life span after menopause.

This recent life extension has led to an enormous amount of confusion. In the 1950s most women who asked for help with symptoms like hot flashes and vaginal dryness were told that the condition was "all in your head." In the mid-1960s, the landmark book *Feminine Forever,* by Robert A. Wilson, M.D., a New York gynecologist, introduced the estrogen deficiency theory. Wilson, no doubt inspired by monies received from drug companies, believed that estrogen was the panacea that could cure any and every menopausal symptom. Were we to believe Wilson, without estrogen at menopause, all women are destined to become sexless "caricatures of their former selves . . . the equivalent of a eunuch." In the early 1970s physicians were routinely dispensing both estrogen and tranquilizers; the combination was probably not only for menopause but also for the trauma resulting from Robert Wilson's book.

In the mid-1970s, however, research studies began to link the use of estrogen in postmenopausal women to increases in cancer of the uterus. There was a decline in its use, which lasted for a few years. Then when newer studies showed that the addition of a synthetic progestin could protect women against uterine cancer, postmenopausal hormone therapy once again became the answer. Even with the documented dangers, in 1990 over 10 million American women were on estrogen-replacement therapy.

Today you can open the Sunday paper and find a two-page ad spread for one of the many estrogen/progestin products on the market. Menopause is big business, and menopausal women have become a prime target market. Unfortunately the health problems that become a greater risk for women at menopause—heart disease, cancer, and osteoporosis —are being linked solely to menopause. This narrow view discounts numerous biochemical, dietary, and lifestyle factors that have been in play for many years of a woman's life, long before menopause, leaving many a female body totally out of balance. This view also disempowers women, implying that they have no control over what is happening to their bodies.

What happens at menopause is explained by the word *menopause* itself. Coming from the Greek, *men pausis,* menopause literally means "month to end," relating to the final monthly menstrual period. The term *menopause* is oftentimes used interchangeably with the more precise term *climacteric.* The climacteric refers to the hormonal changes that start occurring in a woman's body from about the age of 35 and continue to the age of approximately 60. The ovaries, in the course of this natural cycle, dramatically decrease production of the female hormones estrogen and progesterone. While much attention has been given to the role of estrogen deficiency during menopause, the importance of progesterone is often overlooked. Progesterone is one of the body's most important hormones, and has benefits far beyond its role in menstrual cycles and pregnancy, and lack of this essential hormone affects many of our body systems. By making sure our progesterone levels are adequate, we can avoid many of the symptoms of menopause and aging.

The uncomfortable symptoms associated with menopause, such as hot flashes, vaginal dryness, and mood swings, are connected to the lowered hormonal output, but they are not experienced by all women. The more serious health concerns at midlife are also not experienced by all women. So menopause, while occurring universally, is still very much a personal occurrence.

A fact that also needs to be considered is that menopause occurs at a time when the effects of the natural biological aging process are beginning to appear. As we grow older, our bodies do not work the way they did earlier in life, and our poor dietary and lifestyle habits begin to take a heavier toll as we age. This time of life is also often filled with stressful changes for many women: we may find ourselves parenting our parents as they age; our children, who have left home, may be returning home with *their* children; and many women at this age find themselves single either through the death of a spouse or divorce.

After reading everything I could from medical, psychological, social, and emotional viewpoints, I was not relieved, but alarmed. I came up with three major conclusions:

1. Almost without exception, every health problem experienced by women in midlife was somehow blamed on the natural hormonal changes that take place during menopause.

2. The medicalization of this natural midlife process leads to the misconception that menopause is a pathological process and that the problems associated with it (hot flashes, vaginal dryness, osteoporosis, heart disease) are inevitable without medical intervention.

3. The cumulative effects of long-term nutrient deficiencies and negative lifestyle habits, which begin in our teens and continue through our 40s, have been blatantly ignored.

This last conclusion is really the foundation of this book. My research into the whys and wherefores of this life passage began pointing to unbalanced body chemistry as a potent underlying cause of menopausal woes. While about 75 percent of all women experience distressing symptoms purportedly connected to declining estrogen and progesterone, the remaining 25 percent do not suffer any adverse effects. Why? The answer, and perhaps the key solution to menopause, is found in the little-known fact that the reduced amount of estrogen and progesterone from the ovaries is naturally compensated for by hormones produced elsewhere in the body, primarily the adrenal glands and body fat, nature's back-up system. This hidden piece of vital information is a nutritional clue as to why some women suffer through menopause and others don't. When our bodies are overstressed, our adrenals can become exhausted and this natural back-up system fails, leaving us unprotected, and making menopause far more difficult than Mother Nature intended it to be.

Further, this stress on our adrenals may leave many women with progesterone deficiency. Progesterone is necessary for the production of adrenal hormones. When the adrenals are overworked and the hormones it produces depleted, progesterone is constantly used to replenish the system. Progesterone deficiency can cause bone loss, thinning hair, and facial whiskers. Lack of progesterone is particularly common five to eight years before menopause due to the absence of ovulation in many women. An imbalance of the progesterone/estrogen levels creates a condition called *unopposed estrogen dominance,* and excessive amounts of estrogen in the body lead to increased incidence of breast cancer, bone loss, and hypothyroidism.

Dietary habits carried to excess, such as consuming too much sugar and caffeine and following strict fat-free diets, stress our bodies. Caffeine stimulates the adrenal glands, causing adrenaline to be released into the bloodstream. Adrenaline activates our fight-or-flight response, increasing our heart rate, blood pressure, and blood sugar level. When this initial rush wears off, blood sugar drops to lower levels than before the coffee was consumed and leaves the adrenal glands in a depleted state. And then it's time for another cup of coffee. When sugar is added, the problem is intensified, because refined sugars have the same stressful effect on the adrenal glands. In a single day in the United States alone, over 400 million cups of coffee are consumed.

These excessive dietary habits not only lead to adrenal exhaustion that results in damage to our back-up system, but they contribute to other, more serious health problems experienced by women in their midyears. Studies show that women between the ages of 34 and 59 who drink four or more cups of coffee a day have almost three times more the incidence of hip fractures experienced by women who drink little or none at all. And what about soft drinks? The phosphates contained in America's number-one beverage play havoc with calcium absorption. In 1991, 48.4 gallons of soft drinks were consumed per person. The recent popularity of the no- to low-fat diets and the consumption of the wrong kinds of fats—particularly processed oils and hydrogenated fats like margarine and vegetable shortening—led to a nation-wide deficiency of the essential fatty acids. The essential fats make calcium available for the tissues and elevate calcium levels in the bloodstream. And lifestyle habits can't be ignored. Factors like smoking, alcohol use, inadequate exercise, and too much stress also contribute to midlife health problems. Ignoring these lifestyle and dietary factors and focusing on estrogen as the only deficiency is unsound and bad medicine.

When we *have* been given nutritional information regarding disease processes, oftentimes the information is too simplistic and not comprehensive. A case in point is calcium and osteoporosis. We've heard for years that calcium is the singular mineral that builds strong bones and teeth, and that inadequate calcium levels leads to osteoporosis. So we drink our milk and believe we're protected. The latest research suggests that it is not calcium but its overshadowed counterpart, the mineral magnesium, that is the key ingredient not only for strong bones, but for healthy hearts as well. And by consuming too many high-calcium dairy products, we are actually interfering with magnesium absorption. Recent nutritional research also links magnesium deficiencies to a host of conditions that begin to surface in women at midlife; magnesium balance is intimately related with cardiovascular disease, stress, depression, and osteoporosis.

Our health at midlife has its roots in our teens, twenties and thirties. It is during these decades that we need to start taking in enough bone-building minerals, getting enough proper and consistent exercise, and developing positive lifestyle and dietary habits. And yet if we have been neglectful in the past, the uncomfortable symptoms of menopause can become a wake-up call, alerting us to take charge of our own health. Menopause can be a positive motivational factor to make the dietary and lifestyle changes that will ease not only our passage through menopause, but benefit our health for the rest of our lives.

A diet of unprocessed, unrefined, natural foods—including green leafy vegetables, fresh fruits, whole grains, fish, poultry, lean meat, nuts, seeds, and legumes—and moderate amounts of natural and unprocessed oils paves the way to good health. Without proper nutritional reinforcement throughout life, the major glandular changes that take place in our forties and fifties can become medical crises rather than natural transitions.

The problems we associate with menopause are not inevitable. At midlife estrogen levels fluctuate, creating imbalances in calcium, magnesium, and a number of other important minerals and vitamins needed for good health. If imbalances already exist as the result of a lifetime of nutritional neglect, they become magnified by the dramatic glandular changes taking place at menopause, and illnesses like diabetes, hypertension, heart disease, and osteoporosis become greater risks as time marches on.

Although women have been successful in motivating the government to address the virtual lack of research on vital female health problems, the results are a mixed blessing. Menopause is still being viewed as a deficiency disease, and hormone replacement therapy as the panacea for many of the major midlife health threats. In 1990 the federal government initiated the Postmenopausal Estrogen/Progestin Interventions Trial, a 3-year study to evaluate the effects of hormone-replacement therapy on heart disease. In the spring of 1993, the National Institutes of Health announced proposals for new government-funded studies costing an estimated $625 million and running for 15 years. These studies will evaluate low-fat diets, calcium and vitamin D supplementation, and hormone-replacement therapy as preventive approaches to cancer, osteoporosis, and heart disease. Although these studies, with their inclusion of nutritional factors, show promise, their focus on singular dietary or hormone excesses or deficiencies as keys to the prevention of these nutritionally intricate diseases still misses the boat.

We have a great deal of control over how we will respond to menopause by preparing early. Taking an inventory of our eating habits, our weight, our exercise patterns, smoking and drinking history, and heredity factors before menopause occurs will give us some substantial clues to our own journey through this passage. Every woman experiences menopause differently based upon the contents of this inventory. Up to menopause, estrogen provides us with additional protection against heart disease and osteoporosis. After menopause, we are on our own, and the foundation we have laid and our current bad habits—make their consequences known.

On a more positive, preventive note, there are now premenopausal clinics springing up all over the country. These clinics are focusing on women in their mid-thirties and -forties, when estrogen levels first begin to decline, and use a number of screening tools and medical tests to assess a woman's risk of heart disease, osteoporosis, and cancer (cervical, uterine, ovarian, breast), as well as postmenopausal urinary incontinence. By taking advantage of the diagnostic and assessment procedures these clinics have to offer, we can head off potential difficulties. The earlier we take the time to re-evaluate our lifestyles and make meaningful changes, the better our midlife years will be.

It is my hope that this book will empower women, from adolescence to midlife, to begin a nutritional revolution in the way in which we have viewed and treated menopause. Attention to proper diet, exercise, lifestyle changes, and to what the body is saying will make the transition into midlife a time of great freedom and renewed energy. The postmenopausal years should be the best time of a woman's life, when she is freed of child-rearing responsibilities and rewarded with good health. As Margaret Mead put it, "The most creative force in the world is the menopausal woman with zest." Keeping our bodies in biochemical balance is a lifetime adventure that will assure that our passage through each stage of life is filled with zest. The time to prepare is *now*.

1
Menopause:
What It Is, What It Means

Menopause—the end of monthly periods—does not happen overnight. In fact it is a natural transition that occurs over a period of about 15 years, from approximately 35 to 50 years of age. This time frame, known as the climacteric, is characterized by fluctuating hormone levels. It is a time when the production of estrogen and progesterone by the ovaries becomes greatly diminished until the complete cessation of the monthly period. The average age of menopause for American women is 51.

The best predictor of when you will reach menopause is the age at which your mother went through it, because heredity plays a significant role here. Early menopause is more common among black women and southern European or Mediterranean women. Female athletes (especially marathon runners), extremely thin fashion models and women with eating disorders such as bulimia and anorexia, are likely to experience earlier menopause due to lack of body fat and low cholesterol levels. Later menopause is more common among white women of northern European origin. Women from poor socioeconomic conditions reach menopause earlier than those with higher standards of living; women who bear children after age 40 experience a later menopause.

Researchers tell us that if you are a smoker, however, you can reach an even earlier menopause—by three to four years. This is because egg production stops prematurely due to the damage that nicotine and carbon monoxide inflict on the ovaries. They also tell us that strict vegetarians and women with lower than normal cholesterol levels also experience menopause earlier than the average. Other factors contributing to early menopause include having borne no children, being overweight, and having had a late puberty. Women who have had their ovaries removed surgically and are not treated with hormone-replacement therapy are essentially menopausal no matter what their age. Diseases of the pituitary gland and medical irradiation of the ovaries can also induce early menopause.

There are many signals of approaching menopause. Sometimes women will notice two to three years of irregularity in their menstrual cycle, like changes in blood flow and frequency of the monthly period itself. The period may even suddenly go away for months at a time, then reappear. This is why most authorities suggest practicing birth control for at least a year past the last full period. Other signals of approaching menopause include hot flashes and night sweats, vaginal dryness, urinary incontinence, headaches, irritability, insomnia, mood changes, changes in body weight, and loss of sexual drive and interest. Two other hormonally based changes include body-shape changes and altered perception of touch. After menopause, some women may also experience shrinking breasts, thinning hair, and the appearance of facial whiskers due to the loss of progesterone.

All of these signals have been classically and singularly related to the diminishing production of estrogen. The medical approach has been to treat these signals as disease symptoms. Estrogen-replacement therapy (ERT) or, more recently, hormone-replacement therapy (HRT), the combination of synthetic estrogen and synthetic progesterone, are being used routinely as the treatment of choice. These therapies are also being touted as the best way to prevent diseases, such as osteoporosis and heart disease, that become greater risks for women after menopause.

But ERT and HRT are risky. In the 1970s, numerous studies began linking ERT to increases in uterine and breast cancers. In response to these studies, pharmaceutical companies began adding synthetic progestin for 10 days to 2 weeks during the 25-day course of estrogen. While this seems to protect women from risk of uterine cancer, newer studies are showing that its addition may double the risk of breast cancer. The current epidemic of breast cancer in the United States (1 out of 9 women) may very well be linked to long-term use of HRT in postmenopausal women.

Furthermore, there are many women who are definitely not candidates for estrogen or combined HRT. Women at risk are women who have had breast cancer or have a history of it in their families, fibroid tumors of the uterus, heart disease, high blood pressure, blood clots, liver disorders, endometriosis, diabetes, epilepsy, asthma, kidney problems, migraine headaches, and unexplained vaginal bleeding.

We have more empowering choices than just taking hormone therapy or needlessly suffering through the discomforts associated with menopause. A vital and balanced diet, supplemented with vitamins, minerals, essential fatty acids, and herbs that reinforce the body's glandular system can provide natural relief for menopausal discomforts without the known and still unknown risks inherent in hormone replacement therapy. The most common and troubling symptoms of menopause—hot flashes, vaginal dryness, weight gain, heavy bleeding, and depression, irritability, anxiety, and insomnia—can all be helped by the Supernutrition approach.

The Supernutrition Approach to Hot Flashes

Hot flashes are the most common and most distressing menopause symptom. Estimates from various sources maintain that up to 80 percent of all women experience hot flashes at some time during menopause. Hot flashes manifest as a sudden flush of intense heat, often beginning around the neck and face and radiating to other parts of the body. This flushing can bring about episodes of profuse sweating followed by chills. Sometimes when a woman is experiencing a hot flash, her body goes into "overdrive" and her heart begins to beat rapidly. Lasting anywhere from a few minutes to a half hour, hot flashes can be accompanied by dizziness, palpitations, and heavy perspiration. When experienced during the night, these flashes are referred to as night sweats.

There are many theories as to why hot flashes occur. Some claim the lower levels of estrogen experienced at menopause set off a reaction in the hypothalamus, which is responsible for the control of body temperature. Others say hot flashes result from increased levels of hormones secreted by the pituitary gland during menopause. Whatever the hormonal cause, hot flashes occur when there are changes in the diameter of the blood vessels near the skin surface. These vessels dilate, allowing blood to flood into them, bringing heat to the skin surface. Although the skin temperature rises with hot flashes, the body's internal temperature does not rise and there is no fever. While hot flashes can be uncomfortable and annoying, they are not life threatening and do go away, with or without any treatment, once the body adjusts to the lowered estrogen levels.

As we have discussed, the medical profession has generally ignored more natural, less risky methods of alleviating the discomforts of hot flashes. While prescribed estrogen does alleviate hot flashes by artificially maintaining blood levels of the hormone, it does not "cure" them, and in many cases, once therapy is stopped, hot flashes return. The drug clonidine, used for high blood pressure, also has been shown to be helpful for hot flashes, but its side effects include low blood pressure, fatigue, dizziness, and headache.

More natural agents for controlling hot flashes include numerous nutrients and herbs. These substances don't just act to replace something that is no longer there—in this case, estrogen—but I believe they also, specifically, provide beneficial support to the endocrine system, and, in general, improve overall health.

Although many women may be taking multiple vitamin and mineral supplements, at menopause the need for certain nutrients skyrocket. The usual one-a-day vitamin does not meet the requirements of the changing body. For example, the need for vitamin E increases dramatically during menopause, with some women needing 10 to 50 times the usual amount.

Vitamin E has been recognized for its effectiveness against hot flashes for close to 50 years. In research as far back as 1949, vitamin E was found to control severe menopausal flushing in more than 50 percent of the women studied. According to Dr. Evan Shute, a Canadian gynecologist who has been using vitamin E with his patients for the past 50 years, relief from hot flashes can be experienced in a month's use of the vitamin. It is not only helpful in regulating body temperature, but is also protective of the heart (see Chapter 5), improves circulation, and helps prevent varicose veins and blood clots.

With my clients, I recommend starting off at 400 IU (international units) daily, gradually increasing the dosage in increments of 400 IU until symptoms decrease. Many women seem to find relief at levels of 1200 IU a day. A word of caution, however: women who are diabetic or taking high–blood pressure medication or blood thinners should only take vitamin E under their doctor's supervision.

In addition to vitamin E, the bioflavonoids have been found to help minimize the effects and intensity of flushing. These nutrients strengthen capillary walls, have a chemical activity similar to that of estrogen and have been found to reduce the effects of hot flashes when taken regularly; a dosage of 1,000 mg of the bioflavonoid hesperidin has been found to be very effective in alleviating hot flashes. Bioflavonoids, also known as vitamin P, were first identified in the white inner skin of citrus fruits. Food sources include lemons, grapes, plums, black currants, grapefruit, buckwheat, and rose hips. Because the bioflavonoids are often found as companions to vitamin C, it would be wise to choose a vitamin supplement that includes both.

Evening primrose oil, a botanical source of the essential fatty acid GLA (gamma-linolenic acid), has also been used successfully in eliminating hot flashes. Now, I know many of you might be confused about fat. While certain fats are to be avoided, some fats are essential, and must be provided in the diet because the body cannot manufacture them itself. The topic of fat is covered in greater detail in Chapter 5.

Evening primrose oil provides a direct source of GLA, which is essential for hormone production. This essential fatty acid is also necessary for the normal functioning of the reproductive system and the adrenal glands, a source of postmenopausal hormones. In addition, essential fats are helpful in a whole host of hair, skin, and nail conditions, which will be discussed in the next section.

I've been very happy to hear from a number of menopause-age readers who followed my Two Week Fat Flush program detailed in my first book *Beyond Pritikin* (Bantam, 1988), which features unheated, unrefined oil, GLA supplements, protein, vegetables, fruits, fluid, and fiber. They report not only dramatic results with weight loss, but also the cessation of hot flashes and night sweats. I believe this is due to the inclusion of these essential fats in the form of unprocessed vegetable oils and supplements, so necessary for hormonal regulation.

Recently, Japanese researchers have found that a substance known as gamma oryzanol, a naturally occurring component of rice bran oil, dramatically reduces hot flashes. In amounts of 300 mg per day, gamma-oryzanol *caused an 85% improvement in meno-*

pausal symptoms. Maybe the high intake of rice is why Japanese women don't usually suffer from hot flashes.

Herbal remedies work well for some, and many people are more comfortable using herbs simply because they are natural. A number of herbs, including dong quai, ginseng, black cohosh, blue cohosh, hawthorn berries, unicorn and false unicorn root, wild yam root, chaste berry or vitex, and licorice root have been effective in relieving hot flashes. Dong quai, often referred to as the "female ginseng," is the most popular herb used for hot flashes. Siberian ginseng, yam root, black cohosh, licorice root, and dong quai have nontoxic estrogen-like properties that act to balance hormone levels. Care needs to be taken with natural licorice root, as it contains a substance that can lead to fluid and salt retention. The unicorn roots nourish the ovaries, while the hawthorn berries contain many biologically active flavonoid compounds that are capillary strengthening and heart protecting.

Many of these herbs are available individually and in combination in capsule and tincture form at your local health food store. Follow the directions for use printed on the labels. It is very difficult to prescribe exact doses for herbal remedies because every body responds differently. It is important to use common sense and to pay attention to your body's response. You may want to refer to an excellent book devoted to herbs for menopause entitled *Menopausal Years: The Wise Woman Way* by Susun S. Weed (Ash Tree Publishing, P.O. Box 64, Woodstock, NY 12498).

Many women are turning to the homeopathic medical system in addition to herbs. Homeopathy was founded 200 years ago and is currently undergoing a popular renaissance here in the United States. This medical system uses minute dosages of natural substances to stimulate healing. One of the most common homeopathic remedies used for hot flashes is called Lachesis. This remedy, derived from the venom of a South American serpent, has proven effective in cases of severe flushing, night sweats, and headaches. The Pulsatilla homeopathic formula, derived from a perennial herb known as the windflower, can be useful for the more sensitive and emotional woman whose hot flashes are milder in intensity. The Sepia remedy derived from the dried ink of the cuttlefish can be used for the worn out and weakened woman, while sulphur can help the woman who is sleepy during the day and wide awake at night. Homeopathic remedies are generally found in natural food stores. I recommend starting with the lowest potencies like 6×, 12×, 5c, and 7c.

Many women experience relief from hot flashes with the topical use of a progesterone body cream made from natural progesterone extracted from yams grown in Mexico. This natural hormone cream is absorbed through the skin, and carried directly to where it is needed. Unlike the synthetic progesterones, this natural cream is nontoxic and without side effects because it bypasses the liver.

Changing dietary and lifestyle habits can also help in relieving hot-flash discomfort. Use of alcohol, tobacco, and marijuana all negatively affect our hormone levels. Elimination of these substances can do much to make our passage through menopause easier. Consumption of coffee and other hot drinks and of hot, spicy foods, and eating large meals appear to trigger hot flashes in some women. Substituting water or cool fruit juices for hot beverages and eating smaller meals more frequently can help. Our body weight is another key factor in controlling hot flashes.

All of our lives we have been told thin is better, when in fact, a shade on the plump side is really perfect at menopause. Women who are exceptionally thin seem to suffer more during menopause, not only from hot flashes, but from other estrogen-related symptoms as well, since body fat is the prime site of postmenopausal estrogen production. On the other hand, women who are obese may suffer from a constant flow of estrogen being produced by body fat, which can lead to uterine and breast cancer.

The Supernutrition approach gives women the power to regain some control with what is going on with their bodies. Supplements, herbs, and moderation in lifestyle are all things we can use to regulate the changes that naturally occur in midlife. By making healthy choices we can do much to minimize hot flashes and make menopause a more pleasant passage without being at the mercy of doctors.

The Supernutrition Approach to Vaginal Dryness

While you pass through the menopausal years, there will be some changes in your body's sexual response. These changes are due to the effect of decreasing levels of estrogen. Over time, the vaginal walls begin to lose their elasticity and become somewhat drier and thinner. Vaginal secretions become less acidic, and there is more risk of vaginal infections. The mucous secretions from the cervix also decrease, and the vagina itself shrinks, becoming shorter and narrower. The tissues of the bladder and urethra also become more sensitive. This may increase the frequency of urination, with some women needing to void several times during the night. It can also result in increased urinary tract infections, urinary burning, and leaking of urine upon coughing, laughing or sneezing. These changes may cause pain during intercourse and lead us to wonder whether our days of sexual pleasure are over. Luckily there are many things that can be done to help vaginal lubrication.

Small amounts of intra-vaginal Premarin help vaginal dryness, but there are natural choices available other than estrogen. Increased levels of certain minerals and vitamins such as selenium and vitamins A, B, and C help keep vaginal tissue membranes lubricated during and after menopause. Vitamin C is particularly key to the synthesis of hormones in the adrenal glands. The adrenals, two crescent-shaped glands situated atop the kidneys, are designed to produce hormones that are converted to estrogen in body fat when ovarian hormone production slows down. (See Chapter 2, The Forgotten Glands That Manage Menopause, for a more extensive discussion on the role of the adrenal glands during menopause.) Animal studies have shown the need for vitamin C to increase by 75 percent during menopause. So it makes sound nutritional sense to maintain optimal levels of vitamin C—up to 5,000 mg in some cases—during and after menopause. This assures that nature's back-up system (the adrenals/body fat estrogen-producing mechanism) is adequately nourished.

Dietary changes should include increased amounts of vitamin A–rich foods like leafy green and brightly colored orange and yellow vegetables. Vitamin B can be enhanced in the diet by including more whole grains and wheat germ. Vitamin C is found abundantly in citrus fruits, cantaloupe, broccoli, and tomatoes.

Ideally we should be getting most of our vitamins and minerals from food, but modern methods of food growing, harvesting, processing, and transport, as well as environmental stresses from tainted air and water, leave much of our food devoid of essential nutrients. Furthermore, due to hectic lifestyles, fast food, and eating on the run, I recommend women supplement their diets with 25,000 IU of vitamin A or the pro-vitamin A form, beta carotene, and 50 to 100 mg of vitamin B complex daily.

Vitamin E, used both internally and topically, can be used to relieve vaginal dryness. Massaging the inner sides of the vagina with vitamin E oil directly can help heal dry and damaged tissue. Vitamin E suppositories, used once nightly for 6 weeks and then once a week, have proven effective. Additional vitamin E through diet or supplementation is also helpful beginning at levels of 400 IU.

If you find that high dosages of vitamin E are not effective for you, or if you suffer from high blood pressure or take blood-thinning medication—situations where higher amounts of vitamin E are contraindicated—you may want to explore homeopathy. There are three popular homeopathic remedies women can use for vaginal dryness: Lycopodium (vegetable sulphur), Natrum Muriaticum (sodium chloride), and Bryonia (wild hops). Again, I suggest you start with the lower potencies or consult a trained homeopath.

A soothing cream made from the herb calendula is a time-honored remedy used to heal damaged and irritated skin. It has also been used effectively to help vaginal dryness. Calendula cream is available from natural food and herb stores.

A fat-free diet is a dangerous diet, particularly at

menopause. Many of us who are very nutrition conscious and aware of health trends come to menopause with the mistaken belief that all fat is bad. What we may not be aware of, as mentioned earlier in this chapter, is that certain fats are vital to good health! (You may want to refer to my second book, *Supernutrition for Women*, Bantam, 1991, for complete information on the importance of the right fats to female health.) In addition to their significance to hormonal regulation, essential fatty acids are crucial to the cardiovascular, immune, reproductive, and central nervous systems. More specifically, during menopause, deficiencies in these "good fats" are directly related to the drying of vaginal tissue as well as of skin, hair, and nails. Menopausal women suffering from dryness would do well to use oils like flax seed, canola, olive, and sesame seed for cooking and in salad dressings because they provide some of the highest levels of healthy fats.

Avoidance of dehydrating substances, such as alcohol, antihistamines, diuretics, and coffee, and drinking enough clean water (at least two quarts a day) can help with the dryness and itching. Over-the-counter antihistamines and cold pills designed to dry up the nasal tissues can also dry other tissues, including those of the vagina. Use of douches and vaginal sprays should be curtailed, as should use of colored or scented toilet paper, which can irritate sensitive vaginal tissue. Clothes made from natural fibers, such as cotton and silk, are best during this time as they allow the skin to breathe and regulate body temperature, unlike synthetic fibers, which trap heat and moisture next to the skin.

Regular intercourse helps increase the blood flow to the vaginal tissues, which improves tone and natural lubrication. Older women who have remained sexually active throughout their lives seem to have less problems with vaginal dryness. Loving, relaxed foreplay can increase natural secretions, and the use of unscented lubricants during foreplay like baby oil, pure aloe gel, vitamin E oil, or K-Y Jelly can reduce irritation and pain. Natural progesterone cream applied directly to the vagina can help dryness dramatically. A sensitive, patient lover can be a menopausal woman's best friend. Women without sexual partners can use self-stimulation to promote vaginal secretions and reduce dryness.

There are certain exercises that can help increase vaginal blood flow, improve muscle tone, and decrease vaginal dryness. Known as the Kegel exercises, for the gynecologist who developed them, these exercises can be done anywhere at any time. To practice the Kegel exercises, simply imagine you need to stop urinating. Tighten muscles around the anus, urethra, and vagina, hold for the count of three, and then relax.

The Supernutrition Approach to Weight Gain

The preliminary results of a survey conducted by Judith Wurtman, Ph.D., Massachusetts Institute of Technology,[1] seem to indicate that 65 to 75 percent of women involuntarily gain weight at menopause. This weight gain was experienced by women going through both natural and surgically induced menopause, and it appears that a slightly higher percentage of women on hormone therapy gained weight compared to those women who took no hormones. It is interesting to note that these percentages fall into line with the percentages mentioned earlier regarding women who experience difficulty with menopause and those who do not. Those extra pounds that show up at menopause may be due to a lack of progesterone and the consequent estrogen dominance. Estrogen that is not balanced by an adequate amount of progesterone causes weight gain. This is something farmers have known for years, that's why the synthetic estrogen hormone diethylstibesterol (DES) is given to steers to fatten them up. Another reason for the weight gain is that during the first 10 days to 2 weeks of our menstrual cycle, our bodies use up a substantial number of calories in the process of ovulation. So when we stop ovulating (enter menopause) we are left with extra calories, up to 300 daily in some cases, that are not begin burned. Unfortunately, many of these excess calories will end up where we least want to see them if we don't compensate by decreasing our caloric intake or increasing our physical activity. Weight gain during and after menopause may also result from negative attitudes about aging and perceived loss of sexual attractiveness. Many of us choose to compensate for this perceived loss through food. And a lot of the foods that we turn to for comfort—creamy, rich, and sweet—are top-heavy in nutritionally empty calories.

Changing our diets can at times seem overwhelming. A lifetime of eating habits will not be unlearned overnight. You will do well to make your dietary changes one step at a time. A good way to start is by keeping a three-day food journal. This can help to reveal if you are overdoing certain foods (such as fried foods, sugars, and refined, chemicalized and processed foods) and not including enough of others (like fresh fruits, vegetables, whole grains, and proteins from fish, poultry, eggs, and beans). It is important to limit nonessential fats, which are saturated fats found in pork, full-fat dairy products like cheese and ice cream, and the tropical oils such as palm, palm kernel, and coconut. Hydrogenated fats found in margarines and vegetable shortenings function like saturated fats in the body and also inhibit essential fatty acid metabolism, so they should be avoided as well. Increasing vegetables, fruits, legumes, whole grains, and quality protein will help in weight control. The Prime-Time Diet plan in Chapter 8 provides recipes, menu plans, and shopping lists. Remember, it is always important to eat a healthy, balanced diet, but even more so now, to support our bodies as they go through additional hormonal changes.

The Supernutrition Approach to Heavy Bleeding

Fluctuating hormone levels may cause irregular and heavy bleeding in some women during menopause. While heavy, irregular bleeding usually results from the production of too much estrogen and not enough progesterone, other factors, including stress, smoking, alcohol, spicy foods, and caffeine can contribute to it. Fibroid tumors in the uterus can also cause heavy bleeding. The good news is that fibroids are usually benign and most women do not require surgery, as these fibroids will shrink during menopause due to decreased estrogen production. Since uterine and cervical cancer can also cause heavy bleeding, these conditions need to be ruled out. Yearly Pap smears can detect any negative changes in cervical tissue and should be a part of every woman's routine health checkups, even past menopause. A pelvic ultrasound probe called vaginal sonography can uncover fibroid tumors, cysts, thickening of the endometrium, and uterine cancer.

If you suffer from heavy bleeding, there are a number of factors that you can assess yourself. Excessive use of alcohol and frequent use of aspirin both negatively affect the blood's ability to clot and lead to increased blood flow. Lack of exercise can also contribute to heavy menstrual bleeding. Consistent, strenuous exercise lowers estrogen production in the ovaries by inhibiting the production of pituitary hormones. Hot baths or hot showers should be curtailed during periods of heavy bleeding because heat dilates blood vessels, thereby increasing blood flow.

As in all cases of excessive blood loss, iron-deficiency anemia can result. Good sources of dietary iron include red meat, dark green leafy vegetables, beans, and beets. Supplementation with vitamin C or the inclusion of vitamin C–rich foods may be helpful, as vitamin C aids in iron absorption. Increasing the intake of specific iron-rich foods, with accompanying vitamin C, works well for some women. Those who have had chronic, long-term anemia may require more concentrated measures. Supplementation with liquid iron preparations, which are less likely than iron pills to cause constipation, should be considered. If you are not anemic, however, iron supplementation may be unwise. Recent studies have suggested that excess stored iron may increase the incidence of both cancer and heart disease. You may want to request that your nutritionally oriented physician run both a hemoglobin anemia and serum ferritin test. The serum ferritin test is the best way to find out if you are storing excess iron in the body.

Two homeopathic remedies that have been found to stop excessive menstrual bleeding are homeopathic phosphorus and homeopathic belladonna. Many such remedies are sold at health food stores; it is advisable to try the low potencies, such as 6×, 12×, 5c, or 7c first.

The Supernutrition Approach to Depression, Irritability, Anxiety, and Insomnia

Although many women experience mood swings, anxiety, insomnia (sometimes related to hot flashes and night sweats), and depression during the menopausal years, it is important to understand that no psychological disorder has ever been attributed directly to menopause. These symptoms can and do occur in women throughout their lives. Unfortunately, in our culture many women's emotional responses and/or reactions are often blamed on hormones—it's either "that time of the month," or "that time of life." But studies show that when compared with younger women, the menopausal age group shows a significant drop in psychological symptoms. This is not to say that fluctuating hormone levels do not leave many women experiencing correspondingly fluctuating mood swings during this time. These hormone-related mood swings, like the mood swings associated with PMS can throw us for a loop. We may feel out of control, irritable, and anxious. Women need to know they are not going crazy. It is important to remember that although uncomfortable and sometimes frightening, these mood swings are not long term and do go away as the body adjusts to the lowered estrogen levels.

Because there is no one pattern all women go through in menopause, many women really don't know what to expect and describe feeling anxious and out of control. Lack of information about the physical changes they are experiencing can contribute to the intensity of these feelings. Shifting moods and feelings of depression during menopause may result from social and environmental stresses in combination with hormonal changes. Midlife for many women entails many more life changes than just menopause. For many it is a time when children leave home and the focus on child rearing ends. Some women mourn the loss of their ability to bear more children. Unless women have developed their own interests or careers, this change can lead to feelings of personal emptiness. This is also a time when aging parents may need to be taken care of. Some women become widowed, others divorced. Depression is an understandable reaction to the many external life changes that may also be taking place at this time of life.

The prescribing of tranquilizers or antidepressants for menopausal women with anxiety or depression has been common practice for many years. This practice does little to identify or solve the root of the problem, and introduces addictive substances with unpleasant side effects into a body that is already out of biochemical balance, thereby increasing the potential for further physical and psychological problems.

Depression, anxiety, and irritability may also be physically rooted. Fluctuating and declining estrogen and progesterone levels can affect women emotionally, as we have learned from PMS. During menopause, depression and mood swings can be related to the imbalance of estrogen and progesterone. Also, falling estrogen levels affect both calcium and magnesium metabolism, two minerals important for the nourishment and health of the nervous system as well as of bones and the heart (as we will explore in later chapters). Maintaining a healthy calcium/magnesium balance is vital. My research suggests that one part calcium to one part magnesium is recommended. So many menopausal women are taking calcium supplements with no regard to this important biochemical balance. A high intake of calcium without accompanying magnesium can increase magnesium requirements and intensify magnesium deficiency symptoms, such as nervousness, anxiety, and depression.

Good nutrition and supplemental calcium, magnesium, the stress-fighting B vitamins, and amino acids can do much to decrease anxiety and depression and improve our sense of well being. So can eliminating vitamin-robbers like caffeine, alcohol, sugar, aluminum, soda pop, and certain medications like antacids, antibiotics, and diuretics. Exercise, relaxation techniques, and counseling or menopause support groups are other helpful alternatives. There are also a number of herbs including passionflower, skullcap, camomile, and valerian root that can be taken in capsule form, as alcohol-free tinctures, or made into teas. These herbs exert a natural calming effect, relieving anxiety and promoting sleep. Do follow directions on the label.

Cultural Influences

A woman's experience of menopause is heavily influenced by the culture in which she lives. As

Western cultures until now have emphasized youth, beauty, and sexuality as ultimate female standards, it is no wonder that menopause is perceived as a time of loss and regret. With these kinds of cultural attitudes it is not unexpected that many women suffer needless depression at its approach. In non-Western cultures, menopause is viewed much differently. The cessation of childbearing is a positive event in a woman's life, and less attention is focused on physical discomforts. Women reaching menopause are regarded as having reached their peak of power. They are looked on as elders, full of wisdom and experience. Women in certain Native American tribes, for example, gained entry into the Grandmother's Lodge upon reaching menopause. They were respected for the wisdom and power they attained by not losing their "wise blood." Where other cultures make menopause a rite of passage, our culture turns it into a medical event. Women get caught up in focusing on "symptoms," and life often becomes an attempt to "survive" menopause.

However, our culture's attitudes about menopause are beginning to change. As psychiatrist Barry Richmond, Ph.D., of New York's Beth Israel Medical Center puts it, "Our society is not appreciative of older women, at least not yet." As we in the baby-boom generation pass through our forties and fifties, you can be sure that we are not going to respond to the menopause experience with passivity and fear like generations before us. Just as my generation knew PMS was not just "in our heads," but a real biochemical imbalance in the body, we will redefine menopause. Empowered with knowledge about this natural transition, we will be able to support the major glandular changes that take place through the right diet, nutritional supplements, herbs, homeopathic remedies, exercise, and a positive attitude about ourselves. These effective methods of self care will surely gift us with a renewed sense of freedom and energy to take full advantage of the opportunities that await us in the years ahead.

2
The Forgotten Glands That Manage Menopause

When we enter menopause, nature does not simply turn off our estrogen and leave us ready for synthetic hormone-replacement therapy. A natural back-up system, consisting of the adrenal glands and our own body fat, is designed to make up for the declining hormone output. However, the stresses of modern-day living have severely compromised the ability of this secondary system to function.

With the continuing hoopla about hormone-replacement therapy, one important fact has been lost. A woman's body continues to produce estrogen even after menopause, but at lowered, more consistent levels. After menopause, the ovaries continue to produce some estrogen as well as androgens, hormones similar to male hormones. Androgens play an important role in sexuality and health in general. They promote muscle strength, vaginal elasticity, and sex drive. Research has shown that even women in their eighties continue to produce small amounts of androgens.

Androgens are converted to estrogen in the fat of a woman's body, but the ovaries are not the primary source of these important hormones. The adrenal glands produce 80 percent of the androgens circulating in our bodies and used by our body's fat stores to produce estrogen. In essence, a woman's body fat functions like another gland, producing estrogen from raw materials (androgens) and storing it for future release. The amount of estrogen converted in the body's fat is directly related to the amount of body fat present. This is why very thin women (less than 18 percent body fat) seem to have more problems with menopause. Overweight women (more than 25 percent above the ideal weight for their height) have a higher risk of breast and uterine cancer; their body fat is constantly storing and releasing high levels of estrogen for long periods of time.

Androgen-based estrogen protects women from uncomfortable menopausal body changes, but only about 25 percent of women seem to produce enough of this type of estrogen to be able to sail through menopause comfortably. The other 75 percent may be suffering from adrenal insufficiency, exhaustion, or hypoadrenia, a condition in which the adrenals are not capable of meeting all of the demands placed upon them.

Our adrenals are two small glands that are nestled atop the kidneys. These glands are involved in numerous bodily functions, including the manufacture of 28 individual hormones, the digestion of food (especially carbohydrates and sugar), the regulation of the body's minerals, working with the thyroid gland to produce and maintain the body's energy levels, and the synthesis of the hormones adrenaline and noradrenaline in reaction to stress. Progesterone is the primary raw material for producing adrenal gland hormones. When there is not enough progesterone, the adrenal cortex derives its hormone-producing material from a second source, androstenedione. In response, the body manufactures an increased amount of androstenedione, which has a masculinizing effect on women. Thinning hair and facial whiskers may result.

Hans Selye, M.D., a pioneer in the area of stress research, added much to our understanding of the adrenal glands and their functioning. He recognized that stress, no matter what the source, will cause the body to use vitamins and minerals in great amounts, beyond its normal needs. Dr. Selye described what is known as the general adaption syndrome (GAS), noting that stress triggers three distinct stages or reactions.

Stage 1: The Alarm Reaction. In the alarm reaction, the body prepares for stress. The adrenals begin to "hyperfunction," producing extra amounts of hormones to respond to the stress alarm. This is one of the normal functions for which the adrenals were designed. Once the stress is removed, the adrenals quiet down and return to their normal functioning.

Stage 2: The Resistance Stage. If the stress continues for a long period, the body enters the resistance stage. The adrenals begin to adapt by actually increasing their size and function. In order to do this, however, energy will be drawn from the body's reserves. Nutrients not supplied by the diet will be siphoned off from reserve areas. This resistance stage can continue for weeks, months, and even years, until the body weakens due to lack of reserves of both energy and nutrition.

Stage 3: The Exhaustion Stage. In the exhaustion stage, the body's reserves of both energy and nutrition are exhausted. The body can take only so much abuse. The antistress mechanisms are gone and there is nothing left in reserve. This stage of exhaustion, often expressed as fatigue or chronic tiredness, is one of the most common complaints in our culture.

Although we may believe we handle stress very well, stress to our physical bodies comes in many different forms. In addition to the emotional and mental stress we commonly think of, physical stress, including any physical injury, overwork, or lack of sleep, affects the adrenals. Any chemical substance, whether from environmental pollutants or diets high in refined and overprocessed foods, must be detoxified by our bodies, and this, too, puts stress on the adrenal glands. In addition, job stress, lack of or excessive exercise, use of stimulants such as coffee, sugar, and "recreational" drugs, and tumultuous personal relationships contribute to burn-out. Our bodies react in the same manner no matter what produces the stress. Those of us who live with constant, unending worries about finances, children, health problems (either our own or those of someone we love), divorce, etc., use up excessive amounts of nutritional reserves every day, which only adds to the body's overload. And chances are, if we're "stressed out," we're not eating well to begin with.

Early warning signs of adrenal insufficiency include chronic low blood pressure, fatigue, low stamina, sensitivity to cold, and addictions to either sweet or salty foods. Women who consider themselves "night people" often suffer from adrenal exhaustion or burn-out. These women are usually tired when they get up and spend the better part of the day spiking their tired adrenal glands with caffeine, nicotine, sugar, sodas, or excessive exercise. At the end of the day, their burned-out but artificially stimulated adrenals are giving them energy to go all night. This cycle is a red flag for adrenal problems in women.

As you can well imagine, by the time many of us enter menopause, our adrenal glands are either in a state of constant hyperfunction or in burn-out. Hyperfunctioning adrenals can result in many of the same symptoms attributed to menopause itself: high blood pressure, dizziness, headaches, hot flashes, excessive facial and body hair growth, and other masculine tendencies. Adrenal burn-out can also lead to allergies, low blood sugar, and diabetes, which will be discussed in Chapter 6. The chronic mental and emotional stress we live with, combined with poor dietary and lifestyle habits, severely compromise these tiny glands. Not only do they no longer function adequately in response to stress, they are incapable of producing those beneficial androgens that could alleviate many of our menopausal discomforts.

The simplest and best test to identify hidden adrenal burn-out is known as the postural blood pressure test. I believe it is a good idea to have your doctor do this test for you routinely to detect the problem before it is full blown. The test entails the patient being placed in a reclining position for 4 or 5 minutes. The blood pressure is then taken and recorded. A second blood pressure reading is immediately taken and recorded, but this time the patient is in a standing position. The difference in blood pressure levels is the key to diagnosing hypofunctioning adrenal glands. In healthy glands, if the blood pressure drops, the drop is insignificant. When the difference in the two blood pressures is severe, hypoadrenalism is strongly indicated. Blood pressure in individuals with this condition have been known to drop as much as 40 points.

The Supernutrition Approach to Adrenal Support

Our nutritional needs skyrocket at the onset of stress and remain higher than normal during periods of prolonged stress. In the final analysis, whether the stressors come from mental or physical sources, nutrition is the key. We need to fortify our bodies with the extra reinforcement it needs so that our reserves are not depleted. Adequate protein, as well as a number of vitamins, minerals, and herbs, can support and enhance adrenal function during this time.

The minerals in the body are most effected by stress. Magnesium, calcium, zinc, potassium, sodium, and copper are depleted from body tissues as a direct result of stress. Due to the depletion of nutrients from our soils, the very best food sources of naturally balanced minerals come from the sea. Sea vegetables, sold in dried form in health-food stores, provide high amounts of magnesium, potassium, phosphorus, iodine, iron, and other key trace minerals like manganese, chromium, selenium, and zinc. Sea vegetables may not yet be familiar to many Americans, but they should be part of every woman's pantry because of their extraordinary nutrient content. They are also very versatile and can be used as side dishes and condiments. Hijiki, for example, a sea vegetable that tastes a bit like licorice and looks like tangled black strings, contains significant amounts of both iron and calcium. A half cup of cooked hijiki is higher in iron content than two eggs and contains almost the same amount of calcium as that of a half cup of milk. Sea vegetables are also high in protein. Nori, a nutty tasting seaweed that comes in sheets, contains almost 30 percent protein. It can be toasted and crumbled over fish, vegetables, and pasta. I recommend that my clients toast a sheet of nori every morning and crumble it over their whole-grain cereal. In addition to being a good source of minerals, sea vegetables like blue-green algae or spirulina, kelp, nori, arame, wakame, hijiki, and sea palms contain a substance called sodium alginate that pulls toxic heavy metals from the system.

Of course there are more familiar foods that you can choose from. These minerally packed foods include all of the richly colored fruits and vegetables: green vegetables, such as broccoli, collards, kale, and mustard greens; the yellow-orange vegetables, such as squash, pumpkin, carrots, and sweet potatoes; and fruits, such as bananas, strawberries, and cantaloupe. Legumes are rich in iron, soy products like tofu and tempeh are rich in copper, and eggs and meat are good sources of manganese and zinc. Try to purchase foods that are locally grown, which helps to ensure that most vitamins and minerals are not lost in preserving the food for shipping. Labels that certify that the produce was organically grown provide good assurance that no pesticides or herbicides have been used in the growing process.

A surprising number of my clients suffering from adrenal burn-out report strong cravings for chocolate. I find this fascinating because chocolate is a fairly high source of both magnesium and copper, two of the essential minerals which are required for energy production in the adrenals. Chocolate's call may indeed be the body crying for nutrients that have been lost due to stress. Obviously, chocolate, because it contains large amounts of sugar and saturated fats, is a poor choice for magnesium and copper supplementation.

The B-complex vitamins, known as the antistress vitamins, are crucial during stress. Even a slight lack of vitamin B_2 can cause a degeneration of the adrenal glands. Pantothenic acid is essential to the production of many of the adrenal hormones; it also nourishes the adrenals, and a deficiency of this important B vitamin can cause atrophy of the glands. The best sources of B-complex vitamins are desiccated liver, brewer's yeast, legumes, blackstrap molasses, and whole grains. It is important to note that brewer's yeast is high in phosphorus, a calcium-competing mineral, so no more than 2 tbsp. per day is recommended. Food yeast may also be contraindicated in women who suffer from yeast infections.

In addition to the B vitamins, vitamin C, zinc, and manganese are important for healthy adrenal glands. The need for vitamin C has been found to increase dramatically during times of stress, with our bodies needing as much as 2.5 times more than normal. Amounts as high as 3,000 mg are not excessive during times of chronic stress. Vitamin C should be taken in small doses throughout the day rather than all at once, as the body is able to utilize it better in smaller amounts. Vitamin C-rich fruits and vegetables include citrus fruits, cantaloupe, green peppers, and broccoli. A good herbal source of vitamin C is rosehip tea.

Vitamin supplementation can't help if the body is

unable to utilize the nutrients, however. Both manganese and zinc are involved in numerous enzyme systems that are necessary for the absorption of vitamin C and the B-complex vitamins. Deficiencies in these important minerals are prevalent in our diets due to soil exhaustion, overprocessing of foods, careless cooking habits, and the eating of nutritionally empty "junk foods." Good sources of manganese include leafy greens, seaweeds, whole-grain cereals, nuts, and seeds. Good sources of zinc, particularly for women, include lean red meats, eggs, brewer's yeast, seafood, pumpkin seeds, and whole grains.

Herbs can also come to the rescue to help reduce stress, alleviating the strain on the adrenals. Hops, passionflower, skullcap, and Chinese or American ginseng are all beneficial. Numerous studies have shown that ginseng is an "adaptogen," which means it helps the body adapt to excessive stressful states. Hops, passionflower, and skullcap all have the ability to act as natural sedatives, calming the nervous system and relieving headaches and insomnia. These herbs are all available in capsules, nonalcoholic tinctures, and as herbal teas. Another natural aid for stress is the remedy known as Rescue Remedy, made from a combination of distilled flower essences. Used under the tongue or in water, Rescue Remedy is effective for any type of trauma, be it emotional, mental, or physical. It is also available in a cream and can be applied topically to traumatized physical areas on the body.

In addition to nutritional improvements, there are a number of lifestyle changes that can help the adrenal glands recover from exhaustion and help us cope more effectively with stress:

1. Simplify your life. At this time your energy is needed for healing. Cut back on social activities and obligations that create stress and rob you of energy.

2. Take some time every day for relaxation, recreation, and exercise. Initially you may find you have little energy for exercise, so start slow and build up. Be gentle with yourself.

3. Learn to take control of your life and your time. Once we accept responsibility for our lives and stop blaming people and circumstances, we can begin to use our energy to solve our problems.

4. Break the worry habit. The energy wasted worrying can be used in your healing process.

5. Learn to share your feelings, both negative and positive. Join a support group. Learning to release pent-up angers and frustrations can help lessen your emotional burdens.

6. Find something to hit—punch a pillow or hit a tennis ball—to release pent-up emotions.

7. Develop good sleeping habits and make sure your body gets adequate rest.

In the case of the adrenals, many of us would do better if we knew better. Because we have been completely unaware of the existence—let alone the function—of the adrenal glands, we have abused and neglected them through diet and bad lifestyle habits such as ingesting too much coffee, alcohol, and sugar. But given the vital role of the adrenals in back-up hormone support during and after menopause, it is crucial that you make every effort to regenerate these "forgotten" glands, so they can supply the body with adequate levels of estrogen. Maintaining adequate body fat at menopause is also important for assuring healthy estrogen levels. Implementing lifestyle and nutritional changes can do much to nourish the adrenals so that they can function optimally to help ease our transition through menopause.

3
The Calcium Craze

In the last 10 years, women have gone calcium crazy in an effort to prevent brittle bone disease or osteoporosis. In this country sales of calcium supplements surged from $18 million to well over $200 million in 6 short years. Foods from breakfast cereals to canned soups to orange juice are now "fortified" with calcium. Even antacids like Tums are being recommended by some for use as a "dietary" source of calcium.

Why has calcium become such an important health issue? In 1982 Robert Heaney, M.D., a noted bone researcher at Creighton University in Omaha, Nebraska, released his findings of a 15-year study of 200 middle-aged nuns. He observed that those whose diets were low in calcium were excreting more calcium every day than they were taking in. He also noted that low calcium intake put people at risk for osteoporosis, especially older women whose estrogen levels were decreasing due to menopause. Estrogen is especially important in shifting calcium from the bloodstream into the bones. As estrogen levels diminish during menopause, the absorption of calcium by the bone also diminishes, leading to risk of osteoporosis. Dr. Heaney's conclusion triggered an advertising blitz featuring elderly women, hunched over with "dowager's hump," accompanied by the message that calcium would prevent us from ending up in this condition.

Because of this advertising, *osteoporosis,* a disease many of us had never heard of 10 years ago, has now become a household word and calcium supplementation has become big business. Osteoporosis is the result of a negative balance between bone loss and new bone formation. During actual menopause, decreased amounts of estrogen accelerate the rate of bone loss. After three or four years, the rate of bone resorption returns to normal, but osteoporosis will progress if progesterone levels remain low. Progesterone maintains new bone production, and without it the body will not be able to keep up with even normal bone loss.

Hip and back pain, loss of height, and spinal curvature are all signs of osteoporosis. It is a disease that affects more women than men, since men tend to have denser bones to begin with and generally consume more calcium than women. Pregnancy, childbirth, lactation, menopause, heavy dieting, and our addictive dietary and lifestyle habits all challenge the calcium reserves in women, making us more susceptible to this degenerative disease. But calcium supplementation alone is a simplistic solution to a complex situation. Calcium is just one element in a delicate balance of vitamins and minerals our body maintains for optimum health.

Calcium—It's Not Just for Bones

Calcium is the most abundant mineral found in our bodies, and while 99 percent of our bodies' calcium is in our bones and teeth, the other 1 percent that circulates in our blood, fluids, and soft tissues is essential for all life processes. While we all know that calcium gives strength and structure to our bones, we may not know that it also gives these same qualities to every cell in our bodies. Our bodies maintain a delicate balance with calcium. Blood levels must stay between 9 and 11 mg of calcium per 100 cc of blood. When our intake of calcium is too low to maintain this level and blood calcium levels drop, the parathyroid gland releases a hormone that dissolves calcium from our bones to resupply the blood.

In addition to its vital role in forming and maintaining strong bones and teeth, calcium is the key mineral for maintaining muscle tone and elasticity. It is needed for muscle growth, for contraction and relaxation of muscles including the heart, and for prevention of muscle cramping. Recent research has shown that calcium can delay the onset of muscle fatigue and increase stamina. Calcium is also necessary for the absorption of vitamin B_{12}, which keeps our nerves healthy. In addition, calcium works on the nervous system, playing an important role in the transmission of nerve impulses from one part of our bodies to another, "nourishing" the nerves, and exhibiting a sedative effect upon the nervous system. And calcium metabolism has been shown to play a role in ameliorating hypertension, with studies indicating that calcium helps relax smooth muscles of the peripheral blood vessels and therefore can lower blood pressure in certain individuals.[1-3]

Although calcium loss from bone tissue has been identified as a primary "cause" of osteoporosis, simply supplementing with calcium or adding more calcium-rich foods to our diets may not be the best solution. Calcium can only function optimally in our bodies when it is in balance with other vitamins and minerals, especially magnesium. Megadosing with calcium can lead to deficiencies in magnesium, since both minerals compete biochemically for the same receptor sites. Magnesium deficiencies create other health-threatening problems like heart disease. Preventing osteoporosis is not simply a matter of *not* getting *enough* calcium, but of *not absorbing and maintaining* the calcium we do get, and of not keeping it in balance with the other vital nutrients needed for health. The body cannot manufacture minerals so calcium must come from our diet and/or supplementation. Since we have been made aware of our need for calcium through advertising, and so many foods are now being "fortified" with calcium, we may believe that we are getting adequate amounts of this mineral. Indeed, we may be putting more than enough calcium into our bodies, but there are numerous biochemical factors (that the advertisers do not tell us about) that interfere with its absorption.

Our addictive dietary habits and lifestyle choices, including the consumption of sugar, soft drinks, and coffee, severely impedes our body's ability to properly absorb and utilize calcium—and consumption of these three substances has become a national addiction. No matter how calcium-rich our diets are, no matter how much we supplement our diets, if this essential mineral is not being absorbed, it is useless.

Calcium Robbers

Sugar

In order for calcium to be transported to bone marrow, it needs to be in balance with phosphorus. According to Melvin Page, D.D.S., a pioneer researcher in dental endocrinology, the calcium–phosphorus level should be 2.5 parts calcium to 1 part phosphorus. When the balance is disturbed, the bone marrow is starved for calcium, resulting in osteoporosis. Sugar may be the number-one cause of calcium imbalance. This sweet substance, found in so many of our favorite foods, depletes the body of phosphorus, so despite your intake of calcium, if you're eating sugar you're profoundly disturbing the calcium/phosphorus ratio. Without adequate phosphorus for transport, bone marrow doesn't get the calcium it needs, so the body pulls calcium from storage sites in bone. But this cannot be used either without adequate phosphorus. Now there is an "excess" of calcium that cannot be used, so the body excretes it. In the process of being metabolized, refined sugars rob the body of other valuable nutrients, including calcium, magnesium, manganese, chromium, zinc, copper, and cobalt, thereby causing an imbalance in all the body's minerals. This imbalance not only contributes to osteoporosis, but other degenerative diseases as well, including heart disease and diabetes.

Most sources estimate the sugar consumption by the average American to be 120 lbs. per person, per year. Today you will probably eat 30 tsp. of sugar. Although this seems inconceivable to many—and we would not deliberately dip into the sugar bowl and eat 30 tsp. of sugar—that's exactly what you get when you drink a 12-oz. can of Mountain Dew and eat an ice-cream sandwich.

I can hear many of you protesting, "I don't eat sugar anymore. I'm eating more fiber, and I've cut out desserts." But everything, from cigarettes to french fries, has sugar in it. Thirteen tsp. of sugar can be found in low-fat fruit yogurt, and even pickled beets contain almost 10 tsp. per serving. When talking about sugar, we need to understand what we are talking about: sugar is more than the white granulated stuff we put in our coffee. There are more than a dozen other kinds of sugar from a variety of sources, including glucose, fructose, sucrose, maltose, lactose, dextrose, raw sugar, honey, brown sugar, powdered sugar, molasses, maple sugar, corn syrup, high-fructose corn syrup, rice syrup and barley malt. Sorbitol, mannitol and xylitol are sugar alcohols.

These sugars are hidden in an abundant variety of our foods. When "choosy mothers choose Jif" peanut butter, they're also choosing sugar. And if you're eating Lipton Cup-a-Soup, Ritz crackers, Hellmann's mayonnaise, Quaker Instant Oatmeal, Gatorade, bacon, hot dogs, bologna, nondairy creamers, or cream-style corn, you're getting a dose of sugar. Even chewing gum contains one-half tsp. per stick. We pat ourselves on the back for switching from a sugar-coated cereal to Fruit and Fibre, not realizing that it contains 46 percent sugar per half-cup serving. Although much of that sugar occurs naturally in the raisins, malt, and grains, the negative effects of sugar seem to be the same no matter which form you consume.

Food preparers have discovered that sugar is not just for sweetening. Added to foods such as catsup, it helps retain colors; added to baked goods, it ferments yeast and imparts a brown crust to breads and rolls; in soft drinks it adds body and texture; in chewing gum, pliability. Molasses or corn syrup may be added to a restaurant's hamburgers. Raw potato slices are often dipped in sugared water before being fried. Refined sugar, added to air-cured tobacco in the blending process, enhances both flavor and the burning quality of cigarettes.

Supernutrition Ways to Break the Sugar Habit

It would take an entire book to list the food items that contain high levels of sugar. The sad fact is that even those of us who believe we are nutritionally aware are probably getting far more sugar than we need or want. We choose fruit juice over sodas, getting more nutrients but almost the same amount of sugar. We buy fruit juice–sweetened cookies, unaware that the natural juice concentrates used to sweeten them are metabolized by the body in the same way refined sugar is.

Awareness becomes the most important factor in controlling our sugar habit, and reading food labels is the first step. Search for any of the -ose words (*glucose, dextrose, sucrose,* etc.). Sugar will also be listed as corn syrup, honey, molasses, barley malt, or just sweetener. Other suggestions for cutting back on sugar consumption include:

- Make your own muffins, puddings, gelatins, sorbets, and fruit desserts so that you can control the sugar content. In general you can cut back on the amount of sugar called for in a recipe by one-third to one-half without affecting taste.

- Substitute unsweetened fruit juice mixed half and half with mineral water or seltzer for regular or diet soft drinks or just drink 100 percent fruit juice.

- Use fresh fruit as snacks or desserts, but don't go overboard. They are rich in fiber, vitamins, and minerals, but are high in natural sugars.

- Don't use sweets as rewards, either for yourself or your family. More than any other food, sweets become entangled in our psychological and emotional lives; we celebrate with cake, we console ourselves with Häagen-Dazs. Learn your own triggers and work at breaking the habit. Keeping a food diary has been especially helpful for many of my clients.

Soda and Soft Drinks

Sodas are the nation's number-one drink; more soda is consumed than even water. Most sodas not only contain sugar, but they also contain large amounts of phosphoric acid, a phosphorus-containing substance. This is why artificially carbonated drinks used to be called "phospho sodas." They do not, however, contain an equivalent amount of calcium needed to maintain the calcium/phosphorus balance.

While some phosphorus is necessary for bone and calcium metabolism, our diets contain much more phosphorus than calcium. In addition to sodas and soft drinks, phosphorus is found in meat and other protein foods, and in artificially preserved foods. Since the ratio of phosphorus to calcium in our bodies is a critical factor in the optimal use of calcium, drinking soft drinks throws this ratio entirely out of whack. Adding more calcium to the diet would seem to be a way to bring this ratio back into balance. But, at very high intakes, absorption of calcium decreases, while that of phosphorus continues efficiently, and high levels of both have been shown to lead to the loss of other important minerals in the body.[4] So many of us have fallen into a destructive cycle: drinking soda, which depletes our calcium, and then megadosing on calcium supplements in an effort to restore calcium levels, which leads to further loss.

Over the past several decades, our intake of phosphorus has doubled while our calcium intake has declined. Perhaps this is due to the fact that even though we may be taking calcium supplements, we're doing other things that inhibit calcium absorption. Some research suggests that phosphorus from nonessential sources, including sodas and soft drinks and artificially preserved foods, may be more detrimental to the calcium/phosphorus ratio than phosphorus occurring in meat and other protein foods. We would do well to eliminate all sources of nonessential phosphorus from our diets. Certain mineral waters are good substitutes for soda and soft drinks, providing us with additional calcium but no sugar. Six 8-oz. glasses of imported waters such as San Pellegrino and Vittel Grande Source provide 1,200 mg of calcium.

Caffeine

Research shows that calcium as well as other important minerals are lost in the urine due to caffeine consumption. In fact, due to caffeine's diuretic properties, it doubles the rate of calcium excretion. The excretion of calcium stimulates the parathyroid gland to secrete the hormone responsible for drawing calcium from the bone to keep the blood calcium level within normal boundaries. In addition, coffee contains not only caffeine but 29 different acids, and calcium is drawn from bone to neutralize these acids.

Excessive consumption of coffee, tea, regular soft drinks, chocolate, and other foods containing caffeine (see Table 3-1, page 56) will increase your risk for osteoporosis by reducing blood calcium levels, triggering calcium to be pulled from bone, and flushing needed calcium out of your body. When it comes to caffeine, it does not take much to be in excess. A mere three cups of black coffee can result in a 45-mg calcium loss, and women between the ages of 35 and 50 drink more coffee than any other age group.

Caffeine is also found in carbonated soft drinks, (see Table 3-2, page 57) with some studies showing that the combination of caffeine and sugar increases the loss of calcium through the urine more than when either of the two are used alone.[5] In addition to coffee, tea, soft drinks and chocolate, many prescription and nonprescription drugs contain caffeine. According to Food and Drug Administration (FDA) figures, over 1,000 over-the-counter drugs have caffeine as one of their ingredients. These include cold medicines, pain relievers, weight-control products, and allergy remedies. As with sugar, in some cases we are unknowingly ingesting caffeine.

Other Factors Inhibiting the Absorption and Utilization of Calcium

In addition to the "big three," there are other dietary factors that interfere with our body's ability to absorb and utilize calcium.

Table 3-1
Foods and Beverages Containing Caffeine

Product	Caffeine (average mg)
Coffee (5 oz.)	
Brewed, drip method	80
Instant	65
Decaffeinated, brewed	3
Decaffeinated, instant	2
Tea (5 oz.)	
Brewed, major U.S. brands	40
Brewed, imported brands	60
Instant	30
Iced (12 oz.), brewed	70
Cocoa (5 oz.)	4
Chocolate milk (8 oz.)	5
Dark chocolate, semisweet (1 oz.)	6
Baker's chocolate (1 oz.)	26
Chocolate-flavored syrup (1 oz.)	4

Reprinted from *Healthy Bones* by Nancy Appleton, Ph.D. Published by Avery Publishing Group, Inc., Garden City Park, New York. Used by permission.

Table 3-2
Caffeine Content of Soft Drinks

Product	Caffeine (mg per 12-oz. Serving)
Carbonated	
Cherry Coke, Coca-Cola	46
Cherry cola, Slice	48
Cherry RC	36
Coca-Cola	46
Coca-Cola Classic	46
Cola	37
Cola, RC	36
Mello Yello	52
Mr. Pibb	40
Mountain Dew	54
Dr Pepper-type soda	37
Pepsi Cola	38
Carbonated, low-calorie	
Diet Cherry Coke, Coca-Cola	46
Diet Cherry Cola, Slice	48
Diet Coke, Coca-Cola	46
Diet cola, aspartame-sweetened	50
Diet Pepsi	36
Diet RC	48
Pepsi Light	36
Tab	46

Reprinted from *Healthy Bones* by Nancy Appleton, Ph.D. Published by Avery Publishing Group, Inc., Garden City Park, New York. Used by permission.

SAD: The Standard American Diet

The typical American diet is high in fat, sugar, protein, sodium, and phosphorus, all of which cause problems with calcium absorption and utilization. Saturated fats, such as those found in full-fat dairy products such as cheese and ice cream, pork, and beef, and the tropical oils, such as palm, palm kernel, and coconut, combine with calcium in the intestines, forming insoluble compounds and rendering the calcium unusable. On the other hand, essential fatty acids (EFAs) found naturally in cold-water fish, seeds, nuts, and vegetable and botanical oils are essential to make calcium available for tissue use and to elevate calcium levels in the bloodstream. Unfortunately, due to America's fat phobia and penchant for food processing, which destroys EFAs, most diets are lacking in EFAs.

The SAD has been classically high in protein—meat and eggs for breakfast and dairy products, meat, fish, or poultry at other meals. Americans consume more than 100 g of protein a day, two to three times the recommended amount. This excessive amount of protein increases our risk of osteoporosis.[6] High-protein diets create excess nitrogen and sulfur in the blood, which leads to an acid condition. Calcium is leached from bone to neutralize this acid condition and then excreted in the urine. Excess sodium also causes calcium to be excreted in the urine. This in turn lowers blood levels of calcium, signaling the hormone system to cause calcium to be withdrawn from the bones to maintain the proper blood calcium level.

As mentioned above, the ratio of phosphorus to calcium in our bodies is a critical factor in the optimal use of calcium. The typical American diet is low in calcium and high in phosphorus. Too much meat, poultry, nuts, seeds, seafood, whole grains, and soft drinks wreaks havoc with the body's calcium/phosphorus ratio because these foods are much higher in phosphorus than calcium to begin with. Meats such as ham or pork chops contain up to 30 times more phosphorus than calcium; chicken contains more phosphorus (250 mg in 3.5 oz.) than even lean cuts of red meat (158 mg in 3.5 oz. of ground lean beef). High-phosphorus foods, including cow's milk, cause calcium to form insoluble compounds that lead to inadequate absorption of any calcium consumed. Phosphorus is also found in many of the convenience foods we've grown to rely on in our busy lives, like processed cheese, baked goods containing phosphate baking powder, puddings, bread, and instant soups.

Grains

Those of us who follow dietary recommendations for eating a high complex-carbohydrate diet containing heavy whole grains in the form of wheat, rye, oats, barley, and bran may have unwittingly created a calcium-absorption problem. Grains contain phytic acid, a phosphorus-like compound that combines with calcium in the intestine and blocks its absorption. In excess (as in some vegetarian diets), grains can also provide too much insoluble fiber. An over-abundance of insoluble fiber can interfere with the absorption of minerals such as calcium, zinc, and manganese. Fiber binds with these minerals and carries it out of the body, unused.

Oxalic Acid

Excess consumption (on a daily basis) of foods containing oxalic acid can also interfere with calcium absorption. The oxalic acid found in cooked spinach, chard, beet and dandelion greens, sorrel, rhubarb, asparagus, and chocolate bind with calcium to form calcium oxalate, which is indigestible. Some individuals have a tendency to form kidney stones from the calcium oxalate.

Aluminum

Aluminum that is contained in antacids, buffered aspirins, and foods is an unexpected calcium robber. It is estimated that a normal daily intake of aluminum is 20 mg. Many popular antacids (Maalox, Amphojel, Gelusil, Mylanta) contain from 35 to 208 mg of aluminum per tablet. Buffered aspirin, depending upon the particular brand, can deliver an extra 10 to 52 mg of aluminum per tablet. Foods cooked in aluminum pans or wrapped in foil, beverages served in aluminum cans, processed cheeses, cheese spreads, cream cheese, pickled foods, some nonprescription drugs, and peppermint tea all contain additional aluminum. Aluminum-containing antacids, taken three to four times a day for 2 to 5 weeks have been shown to inhibit absorption of phosphorus. While too much phosphorus creates a problem with calcium utilization, too little phosphorus is just as detrimental. Too little phosphorus leads to a decrease in the absorption of calcium from the gastrointestinal tract and the excretion of calcium in urine and feces, especially in individuals with low calcium intake.[7]

Lack of Hydrochloric Acid

Most of the calcium in foods and supplements is in the form of insoluble salts. These salts depend on an acid pH in the stomach in order to dissolve and become bioavailable. Normally, the hydrochloric acid in our stomachs creates this acid pH, dissolving the calcium and breaking it down so it can be absorbed into the blood. But a lack of hydrochloric acid, a condition known as *achlorhydria,* seems to be a common problem in women over the age of 50, putting them at risk of calcium absorption problems.[8-10] Symptoms of achlorhydria include intestinal or stomach gas and bloating after meals. Achlorhydria may be the result of drinking liquids with meals, chewing too little, or eating too fast. Recent research has also shown that people with type A blood have a genetic predisposition to achlorhydria.

Many people who develop stomach or digestive problems begin to treat themselves with over-the-counter antacids, believing that these problems are the result of too much stomach acid. All antacids reduce the hydrochloric acid in our stomachs, thereby interfering with calcium absorption, and, as noted earlier, many contain aluminum, which inhibits the absorption of phosphorus and increases the excretion of calcium. And while Tums is being touted as a good source of calcium, it contains no magnesium, which is necessary for calcium absorption. Ironically, Tums is specifically designed to reduce the very stomach acid needed to enhance the absorption of the calcium it contains. The calcium in Tums rarely gets out of the gut and into the body.

So Where Do We Get Our Calcium?

Now that you've given up coffee and soda, cut down on your sugar and protein, where are you going to get your calcium? The dairy industry has not been shy in telling us that dairy products contain abundant calcium. The vast majority of us grew up knowing that milk builds strong bones and healthy teeth. Indeed, most of us were raised on milk and still look to it and other dairy products as good sources of calcium. And yet we as a nation consume more dairy products than any other, and still have more calcium-related degenerative diseases, including osteoporosis, osteoarthritis, arteriosclerosis, and cataracts, than nations where dairy consumption is minimal or nonexistent. In Asia and Africa, areas where milk products are not included in the diet, the incidence of osteoporosis is negligible, while in Europe and North America, where milk and milk products are heavily consumed, osteoporosis is reaching epidemic proportions.

To Drink or Not to Drink— Milk, That Is

It is true that milk is rich in calcium—1,200 mg per quart to be exact, more than enough to satisfy a whole day's requirement. It is also almost equally rich in phosphorus, the mineral that we have already discussed that has that biochemical bad habit of interfering with calcium absorption. Due to milk's high phosphorus content (the ratio is 1.2 parts calcium to 1 part phosphorus), calcium absorption is impaired. Infants drinking mother's milk, which contains only 300 mg of calcium per quart but has a beneficial calcium/phosphorus ratio of 2:1, actually absorb more calcium than infants drinking cows' milk.[11] Milk and milk products also tend to neutralize hydrochloric acid in the stomach and generate excessive mucus in the intestines. Both of these factors also interfere with the proper absorption of calcium.

Another factor in calcium absorption is magnesium. While magnesium helps calcium absorption, too much calcium interferes with the absorption of magnesium. Magnesium reduces the body's need for calcium, but calcium increases the body's need for magnesium. Although this may seem confusing, humans evolved in a magnesium-rich, calcium-poor environment. Our bodies, therefore, learned to conserve calcium but not magnesium. Even now it makes good sense to favor magnesium-rich foods in our diets. But milk has 10 times more calcium than magnesium. It would be wise to limit this "perfect food" for the perfect calcium/magnesium balance.

For the majority of the world's adult population, milk is a source of calcium they cannot biochemically utilize. At some point between the ages of 18 months and 4 years, most people stop producing the intestinal enzyme called lactase that is needed to break down milk sugar, or lactose. This normal process is similar to that of the animal world, where the lactase enzyme becomes unnecessary shortly after weaning. The resulting lack of lactase causes undigested lactose to move into the colon, where it ferments, resulting in bloating, gas, cramps, and, in some cases, diarrhea. Humans are the only animals that continue to drink milk after weaning, yet worldwide, far more people suffer from lactose intolerance than do not, and therefore cannot benefit from the calcium in milk (see Table 3-3, page 65).

While advertisers have focused our attention on the calcium in milk, they have neglected to honestly inform us about its fat content. The fat content in milk is saturated fat, which has been implicated in cardiovascular disease. The milk industry deceptively reports fat content by weight rather than by calories, so that while whole milk is labeled 3.5 percent fat by weight—which seems acceptable—49 percent of its calories actually are from fat—which is outrageous. Skim milk, which is indeed low in fat (2 percent fat calories), ends up to be a highly concentrated protein because when the fat calories are removed, what is left is mainly protein. As mentioned previously in this chapter, too much protein in our diets leads to calcium leaching, so even skim milk is not a good alternative source for calcium.

Nondairy Sources of Calcium

There are numerous foods rich in calcium and balanced in their phosphorus levels. More calcium can be found in a cup of cooked collard greens than in a cup of milk, and two tbsp. of good old-fashioned blackstrap molasses has almost the same amount of calcium as a cup of milk. Many individuals use soy products as dairy substitutes. It is important to remember, however, that if you are using tofu, the cheeselike soybean curd, as a source of calcium, it is calcium-rich only when calcium sulfate has been added for coagulation. Similarly, soy milk, unless it has been fortified with extra calcium, is not a substantial calcium source. Interestingly, although chocolate is calcium deficient, one-quarter cup of carob flour, a healthy chocolate substitute, contains a respectable 120 mg of this bone-building mineral. Herbs rich in calcium include nettle, comfrey, dandelion greens, watercress, chickweed, and seaweeds such as hijiki,

Table 3-3
Statistics of Lactase Deficiency

Population Group	Prevalence of Lactase-Deficient Healthy Adults (%)
Filipinos	90
Japanese	85
Taiwanese	85
Thais	90
Indians	50
Peruvians	70
Greenland Eskimos	80
American blacks	70
Bantus	90
Greek Cypriots	85
Arabs	78
Israeli Jews	58
Ashkenazi Jews	78
Finns	18
Danes	2
Swiss	7
American whites	8

(From Oski, FA, M.D.; *Don't Drink Your Milk.* Mollica Press, Ltd., Syracuse, NY, 1983.)

wakame, and kombu. A half cup of cooked hijiki is almost as high in calcium as a half cup of milk.

Table 3-4 gives you many other choices for your daily diet.

Increasing calcium absorption, rather than merely increasing calcium levels in our diets, is sadly overlooked in our quest for strong bones. Also overlooked is the bone-building team of vitamins and minerals, whose balance is as important as calcium for the health of our bones. When we upstage the other essential elements by increasing only our calcium levels, we court disaster by disrupting our biochemical balance and putting ourselves at risk of other health problems such as atherosclerosis and kidney stones. The next chapter will introduce you to the rest of the team.

Table 3-4
Nondairy Calcium Sources

Food/Substance	Mg/100 g Edible Portion (100 g = 3.5 oz.)
Kelp	1,093
Carob flour	352
Dulse	296
Collard leaves	250
Turnip greens	248
Barbados molasses	245
Almonds	234
Brewer's yeast	210
Parsley	203
Corn tortillas, lime added	200
Dandelion greens	187

Food/Substance	Mg/100 g Edible Portion
Brazil nuts	186
Watercress	151
Goat milk	129
Tofu	128
Dried figs	126
Sunflower seeds	120
Wheat bran	119
Buckwheat, raw	114
Sesame seeds, hulled	110
Ripe olives	106
Broccoli	103
English walnut	99
Spinach (raw)	93
Soybeans, cooked	73
Pecans	73
Wheat germ	72
Peanuts	69
Miso	68
Romaine lettuce	68
Dried apricots (unsulphured)	67
Rutabaga	66
Raisins	62
Black currants	60
Dates	59
Green snap beans	58
Globe artichoke	51
Dried prunes	51
Pumpkin and squash seeds	51
Cooked dry beans	50

(Data from Endo-met Laboratories, Phoenix, AZ, based on evaluation of existing literature.)

4
Osteoporosis

More than 25 million American women suffer from osteoporosis. Every year as many women die from osteoporosis-related injuries such as hip and spinal fractures as die from breast cancer. In fact, every year there are 1.3 million fractures that result from this bone-thinning disease. Since 1941 when it was first identified as a disease, osteoporosis has become a widespread, expensive public health problem, with health-care costs exceeding $10 billion annually. Osteoporosis is not simply a "calcium-deficiency disease." It is a complex condition that develops slowly over a period of years before it reaches the stage where it can be diagnosed. Unfortunately, it is often a difficult problem to diagnose until it is too late. For this reason, women should take note of early osteoporosis warning signs, such as periodontal disease, changes in the curvature of spinal column leading to "dowager's hump," or unrelenting back pains.

Standard x-rays can only detect bone loss after it is in an advanced stage. There are now more sensitive screening tests available that can more accurately predict the early onset of osteoporosis. Single-photon absorptiometry (SPA) measures bone density in the wrist. Another test, called dual-energy x-ray absorptiometry (DEXA), assesses spinal and hip-bone density. If both of these tests show lowered density, additional blood and urine tests generally are called for.

In order to understand this disease, we need to understand some things about our bones themselves. First of all bone is living tissue made primarily of calcium, but also of other essential minerals and protein. There are two types of bone in our bodies: *compact bone* which is found in the shafts of long bones because it is able to withstand tensile stress, and *trabecular* or *spongy bone,* which is more weight efficient and is found in heel bones, vertebra and at the end of long bone shafts. Compact bone looks solid and hard, while spongy bone is like its name, spongy and filled with holes. Within both types of bone are two groups of bone cells; one type, osteoclasts, breaks down old bone and the other, osteblasts, is responsible for making new bone. This breaking down and rebuilding process is called *remodeling* and takes place throughout our lifetime. The "turnover" time for compact bone is approximately ten to twelve years; the "turnover" time for trabecular bone can be as short as two to three years.

Anywhere from 5 to 10 percent of our bone is replaced every year by this remodeling process. From childhood until our early twenties, depending on sex, race, exercise levels, nutrition, and overall health, bone is made faster than it is broken down, resulting in the formation of dense, healthy bones. According to the peak bone mass concept,[1,2] by our early twenties our bones reach their peak of perfection. The greater the bone mass we achieve by this point in our lives, the less our risk of osteoporosis. Therefore, prevention of this crippling disease begins in childhood and adolescence with proper nutrition for strong healthy bones.

By our late thirties and early forties, the balance of bone growth and loss begins to change and a slow, steady decline in total bone mass begins. Age-related bone loss seems to be normal, but rapid or accelerated loss of bone results in osteoporosis. Bones become weakened and brittle; the walls of compact bone become thinner and softer, and the holes in the spongy bone become larger, leading to a greater risk of fractures and breaks. While the rate and amount of bone thinning varies widely among individuals, generally among women bone loss begins in their mid-twenties and accelerates 4 or 5 years after menopause.

The Question of Estrogen

While advertising is beating us over the head about calcium, doctors are routinely prescribing estrogen to pre- and postmenopausal women for prevention and/or treatment of this complex condition. Estrogen restrains osteoclasts and thus slows bone resorption. With menopause, the decline in estrogen allows osteoclasts to increase the rate of bone loss, thus accelerating osteoporosis. Estrogen is also important in shifting both calcium and magnesium from the bloodstream into the bones. As estrogen levels diminish during menopause, the absorption of these critical nutrients by the bone also diminishes. However, while lowered estrogen levels during and after menopause are a factor in bone loss, I question the routine prescribing of estrogen to treat or prevent osteoporosis, when there have been no definitive studies showing that lower levels of this hormone *cause* this condition, and because just as much bone is lost when estrogen therapy is interrupted or stopped as would have been if it had never been started.[3] Common medical practice ignores the fact that many other factors, including past and present amounts of calcium and other bone-building minerals and vitamins in the diet, an individual's ability to absorb these important nutrients, past and present exercise levels, and dietary and lifestyle habits contribute to the risk of developing osteoporosis.

An apt analogy can be made with an automobile. When a car begins using too much oil, we know better than to blame the oil. Lack of proper maintenance, regular oil changes, and tune-ups over the years has led to this problem. We can continue to drive the automobile and pour oil into it to keep it functioning and risk further damage by just treating the symptom, or we can take it to the auto mechanic and get to the root of the problem. Perhaps we'll need a complete engine overhaul, a balancing, if you will, of the pistons, rings, and valves. Similarly, if we have carefully maintained our bodies over the years with proper diet and exercise, our bodies will be in balance and our declining estrogen levels will not create the severe problems we have been told to expect. Adding more "oil" in the form of estrogen will not cure the problems and may put us at greater risk of other, more serious health problems.

Prevention is the key to maintaining healthy bones and avoiding crippling fractures in our later years, and prevention of this complex disease is a lifelong process that involves far more than simple calcium supplementation or estrogen replacement therapy alone. We need to rely more on a good, balanced diet and make healthy lifestyle choices to maintain not only strong, healthy bones, but also our general health and our body's balance.

The Progesterone Connection

The role of progesterone and its connection to osteoporosis has been grossly overlooked. One of the major physiological effects of progesterone is to stimulate new bone formation. This is particularly important during menopause, when decreased estrogen levels cause rapid bone loss. Unfortunately, many women arrive at menopause with a profound progesterone deficiency, due to adrenal exhaustion. Natural progesterone body cream may be quite helpful in restoring hormonal balance to the system before menopause occurs, thereby preventing bone-thinning.

Not By Calcium Alone: The Bone-Building Nutrient Team

Bone is more than just calcium, and it takes more than just calcium to keep it healthy. Bone is an active, living tissue that has nutritional requirements for optimal health. Because so much attention has been given to calcium and estrogen in the treatment and prevention of osteoporosis, the role of many of the following vitamins and minerals—essential for bone strength and integrity, as well as for adequate absorption and utilization of calcium—has been ignored. Also ignored is the fact that our diets are lacking in many of these essential vitamins and minerals. This lack is due in part to the depletion of minerals in our soil. The advent of "modern" agricultural farming methods has left us with a legacy of poor soil, poor food, and consequently poor health. Eating over-processed food and making poor dietary choices also play a major role in deficiencies of basic vitamins and minerals.

Magnesium

With all the focus on calcium for building strong healthy bones, the significance of magnesium has virtually been ignored, and yet it is a key mineral in healthy bones. Although bone is only 0.1 percent magnesium, the interaction of calcium and magnesium is a vitally important one. Magnesium is essential to help balance and complement calcium and phosphorus. It is vital for calcium metabolism and helps transport calcium from the blood into bone and soft tissues. Magnesium also helps prevent formation of calcium oxalate crystals (kidney stones), and it is needed to convert vitamin D to its active form so that calcium can be absorbed into the bone. Calcium and magnesium must be in the proper ratio to one another to work effectively. When the recommended 1:1 calcium/magnesium ratio is exceeded in favor of calcium, magnesium deficiency can sometimes result. Magnesium deficiency symptoms may include nervousness, irritability, depression, fatigue, palpitations, tremors, spasms, and irregular heartbeat. Magnesium deficiencies have been shown to lower both blood calcium and cholesterol levels, in turn lowering the availability of calcium for bone and affecting the metabolism of estrogen, as cholesterol is the raw material for the estrogen hormone.[4,5]

Magnesium is depleted from our bodies by excessive consumption of highly processed foods, alcohol, birth control pills, and stress. Magnesium deficiencies are common in the American population as a whole and in osteoporosis patients specifically.[6] Menopausal women who are supplementing their diets with 1,000 mg or more of calcium may be inadvertently creating a greater magnesium deficiency, because these increased levels of calcium increase the demand for the already deficient magnesium. This situation can lead to numerous health problems, including the very one which the addition of calcium was intended to prevent. For this reason, a heavy intake of dairy products should be avoided; these foods have up to 10 times more calcium than magnesium. Also make sure you do not take your calcium supplement with a magnesium supplement. If taken together, the calcium can negate the magnesium, rendering it useless.

Although the recommended daily allowance (RDA) for magnesium is 400 mg, the typical American consumes less than 100 mg per day.[7] Americans typically do not favor foods that are high in this essential mineral. Magnesium-rich foods, such as leafy green vegetables, kale, celery, alfalfa sprouts, beans, seeds, and nuts, are often passed over for more processed foods and snacks that are low in magnesium. In addition, our favorite drinks, including coffee, tea, colas, and alcohol, wash magnesium out of the body through the urine.

Vitamin D

The body also needs vitamin D to move calcium from the digestive system into the bones. Vitamin D is made in the skin, with the help of the EFAs, in the presence of sunlight. Normally, daily exposure to sunlight for as little as 20 to 30 minutes provides enough vitamin D for our bodies. Low vitamin D levels are common in older women because as we get older, the body is less able to manufacture vitamin D from exposure to sunlight. Furthermore, if women are not taking in some vitamin D–fortified milk, breakfast cereals, sardines, tuna, sweet potatoes, yams, alfalfa, or egg yolks, deficiency will result. Vitamin D requires conversion by the liver and kidneys into its activated form, so individuals with liver or kidney problems may experience difficulties with vitamin D absorption. Deficiencies of Vitamin D result in bone disorders, such as rickets in children and osteoporosis in adults. Due to the vitamin's effect on the eye muscles, deficiencies may result in nearsightedness. Loss of calcium from the bones in the ear can result in a loss of hearing. The RDA for vitamin D is 400 IU.

Vitamin C

Vitamin C is essential for the formation of collagen, the major structural component of bone. Studies show that a lack of vitamin C may contribute to osteoporosis.[8] Although probably one of the most well-known vitamins, studies and surveys still report deficiencies of this important nutrient, especially in older people. The RDA for vitamin C is 60 mg, but remember that vitamin C needs are increased by all kinds of stress, and it may be beneficial to consider supplements of 2 to 4 g per day during menopause. Natural vitamin C is found in citrus fruits, such as grapefruit, oranges, lemons, limes, cantaloupes, pineapples, and strawberries. Vegetables such as tomatoes, red and green peppers, cabbage, Brussels sprouts, and parsley are also rich sources of vitamin C.

Boron

Researchers at the U.S. Department of Agriculture (USDA) recently found that after 8 days of 3-mg supplements of boron, the postmenopausal women studied lost 40 percent less calcium, 33 percent less magnesium, and slightly less phosphorus than those not taking the supplements.[9] Finding double the prestudy blood levels of the most active form of estrogen, researchers concluded that boron is necessary for the synthesis of estrogen and vitamin D. A recent study showed that supplementation of boron raised serum estrogen levels of postmenopausal women not on estrogen therapy to levels comparable with women receiving estrogen replacement.[10] There currently is no specific RDA for boron, but it is suggested that 1 to 2 mg of boron a day can meet the body's needs. Boron is an essential trace element, meaning it is essential to our well-being, but we only need small amounts of it each day. Boron is found in plant foods, especially fruits (fresh or dried), vegetables, nuts, and honey. Table 4-1 lists the boron content of some common foods.

Manganese

As previously discussed, manganese is essential for the utilization of vitamins B and C in keeping our adrenal glands healthy. This trace element is also needed for the synthesis of cartilage and other connec-

Table 4-1
Boron Content of Foods

Food	Boron Content (mg)
1 medium apple	1
$1\frac{1}{2}$ cups apple sauce	1
$2\frac{1}{2}$ cups grape juice	1
1 g prunes (unsulphured)	27
1 g raisins (unsulphured)	25
1 g dates (unsulphured)	9.2
1 g almonds	23
1 g peanuts	18
1 g hazelnuts	16
1 g honey	7.2

(Based on evaluation of existing literature.)

tive tissue, and for bone growth and maintenance. In a comparison of blood and bone samples of women with osteoporosis and women of the same age without osteoporosis, manganese levels in women with osteoporosis were 75 percent lower.[11] At least half of the manganese in the diet is lost when whole grains are replaced by refined flour. Foods high in phosphorus and calcium, bran, and other high-fiber foods also tend to deplete manganese, so it is prudent to ensure your intake of this vital mineral through supplementation. The RDA for manganese is from 2 to 5 mg. The best food sources of manganese are mainly vegetarian sources such as nuts, seeds, whole grains, seaweed, and dark leafy greens.

Vitamin K

Vitamin K is produced in the body by our friendly intestinal bacteria. Best known for its blood clotting action, vitamin K is also needed to produce osteocalcin, a protein substance found in large amounts only in bone and from which calcium is made. Without sufficient vitamin K, the body does not manufacture enough of this bone-building material, and without osteocalcin, calcium does not crystalize and leaves bone soft and weak. Vitamin K also reduces the amount of calcium lost in the urine, sometimes by as much as 50 percent,[12] and it also speeds the healing of fractures, apparently by stimulating bone growth.[13] Levels of vitamin K in osteoporotic patients have been found to be one-third the normal amount.[14] Vitamin K deficiency is seen in individuals who use antibiotics frequently, as they destroy our friendly intestinal bacteria. The RDA for vitamin K is approximately 65 IU for women. Dark green leafy vegetables, alfalfa, and kelp are rich sources of vitamin K. Yogurt, egg yolks, fish-liver oils, and milk are also good sources.

Zinc

Our skeletons contain most of the zinc in our bodies. One hundred different enzymes, most of which are related to cell growth and health, need zinc as a cofactor. Zinc is vital for normal bone formation and enhances the biochemical actions of vitamin D, which is vital in absorbing and transporting calcium. As important as this trace mineral is, zinc deficiency is common in America. One recent dietary survey reported that 68 percent of adults in this country consume less than two-thirds the recommended level of zinc.[15] This is quite possibly due to the fact that 22 of the 50 states have soils that are deficient in zinc and therefore produce foods that are deficient in zinc. Food processing also removes zinc. Add to this the fact that zinc-rich foods such as red meat and eggs are being avoided because of misguided cholesterol concerns, the popularity of unbalanced fad diets, and the great amount of stress people experience today, and you're left with a zinc-deficient nation. The RDA for zinc is 12 mg. Good sources of zinc include eggs, meat, seafoods, pumpkin seeds, whole-grain cereals, dried beans, and legumes. Particularly oysters.

Copper

Copper deficiencies result in reduced bone strength and mineral content. Copper is essential for the production of lysyl oxidase, an enzyme integral in the formation of collagen, a body protein that provides the basic material for the connective tissues, cartilage, and bone. In today's environment, few women are technically deficient in copper. Rather, they are actually copper toxic because of excessive copper accumulation in the brain, liver, and other organs. When it accumulates in the tissues, copper becomes bio-unavailable and cannot fulfill its role in bone building and maintenance. Copper imbalances result from zinc and molybdenum deficiencies and environmental copper exposure (water pipes, cookware, birth-control pills, and dental materials). There is no established RDA for copper; most nutritionists, however, recommend from 1.5 to 3 mg copper per day. The richest dietary sources of copper are organ meats like liver, seafoods, nuts, seeds.

Silicon

Although little is known about this element and its role in human health, silicon does promote the formation of bones and teeth, and high amounts are found at calcification sites in growing bones. Silicon makes firm, strong tissues, and is contained in collagen. Since the mineral is lost so easily in food processing, supplementation may be necessary. There is no RDA for silicon. It is found in the highest amounts in the hulls of wheat, oats, and rice, in alfalfa, and in the herbs comfrey, nettles, and horsetail.

Vitamin B_6 (Pyridoxine)

Like copper, vitamin B_6 is a cofactor for the enzyme lysyl oxidase. Lysyl oxidase strengthens connective tissue by cross-linking collagen strands. B_6 also is instrumental in the conversion of the toxic amino acid homocysteine to a nontoxic form, cysteine. Homocysteine can interfere with collagen synthesis and therefore jeopardize bone strength. Sources of vitamin B_6 are brewer's yeast, bananas, carrots, onions, asparagus, peas, sunflower seeds, walnuts, and wheat germ. The RDA for B_6 is 1.6 mg; I recommend up to 200 mg per day for menopausal women.

Folic Acid

Folic acid is another nutrient that can disarm homocysteine. Our body's ability to change homocysteine into a nontoxic derivative seems to decrease at menopause, and studies show that folic acid can prevent high levels of homocysteine in postmenopausal women.[16] Folic acid is another nutrient that is often deficient in the American diet owing to food processing and preparation. The best sources of folic acid are the green leafy vegetables, such as kale and chard, that are not dietary favorites of most Americans. Folic acid is also manufactured in intestinal bacteria, so a history of antibiotic and oral contraceptive ingestion can mean a depletion of the folic acid–making bacteria in our intestines. Use of tobacco and alcohol also lead to a deficiency in this important B vitamin. The RDA for folic acid is 400 μg. Higher amounts are available only by prescription. Other sources of folic acid include tuna, salmon, cheese, brown rice, beef, beans, and barley.

Risk Factors for Osteoporosis

Living to a ripe old age is sure to result in some loss of bone tissue. But not everyone—and not even every woman who goes through menopause and lives with reduced estrogen levels—develops osteoporosis. Certain heredity factors have been identified that increase the likelihood of developing osteoporosis; these are things over which we have no control.

While both men and women develop osteoporosis, women are at greater risk. Women's bones are lighter and smaller, and a greater proportion of their total bone is lost as compared to men. Women are also at greater risk because bone loss occurs much more rapidly as estrogen levels decrease. The earlier the onset of menopause, the greater the risk of developing osteoporosis due to reduced levels of estrogen for a longer period of time. Women who are thin, short, and have a small frame and small bones are more at risk. These women have less body fat stores and therefore produce less estrogen after menopause than heavier women.

Osteoporosis is more common among whites, especially of northern European extraction, and Asians. Black women have a lower risk because their bones are normally larger and they lose bone mass more slowly. If you have a mother, grandmother, sister, or aunt who develops osteoporosis, you are more likely to develop it, too. Also, certain diseases, including endocrine disorders, diabetes, and arthritis, put you at greater risk.

In addition to these hereditary factors, there are certain lifestyle habits that increase your risk of developing osteoporosis. These things we *do* have control over, and we need to take steps to change if we want to live a long and healthy life.

Medications

While some medications are necessary and prescribed by your doctor, excessive use of certain drugs may lead to osteoporosis due to calcium loss. Diuretics like Lasix, corticosteroids, excess thyroid medication and prolonged antibiotic use often deplete the body's store of calcium. If you are currently taking any of these medications, you should take extra steps to ensure that your calcium level is maintained.

Excessive Use of Alcohol

It is believed that alcohol suppresses the growth of new bone by poisoning bone-forming cells. In addition, alcohol has an extraordinarily negative effect on the ovaries, causing hormonal imbalances. Nutritional problems resulting from heavy alcohol use include irritation of the intestinal lining, leading to a decrease in absorption of nutrients, and liver damage, which interferes with the production of vitamin D, both of which problems will inevitably effect the development of strong bones.

Smoking

Smoking more than doubles a person's risk of developing osteoporosis. Smokers often carry high levels of the toxic mineral cadmium in their blood, and one well-known result of high cadmium levels is a loss of calcium from bone, resulting in osteoporosis. Researchers also believe that smoking interferes with estrogen production and the way the body handles this hormone. Smokers have decreased blood and tissue levels of estrogen, and smoking leads to earlier menopause, leaving the body with lowered levels of estrogen for a longer period of time.

Lack of Exercise

Exercise increases the amount of calcium in the body because it jars the skeleton, and bone growth and calcification is stimulated by the mild electrical charge from the stress exerted. Conversely, bones lose calcium during inactivity. The familiar adage "use it or lose it" certainly applies to bones. Healthy bones maintain their strength also by having muscles pull on them. Bone mass increases or decreases in direct proportion to the demand put on it. Weight-bearing exercise has been shown to be the best physical activity for increasing bone mass. Exercise gained through walking, jogging, dancing, playing tennis, jumping rope, lifting weights, and playing racquet sports is good for preserving bone. Swimming puts only minimal stress on the body and so does not qualify as weight-bearing. But balance is the key here, for too much strenuous or vigorous exercise can have a negative effect, lowering body fat levels to the point that estrogen production is interfered with, thereby effecting calcium absorption. Lowered body fat is also tied to irregularities in menstruation. Richard A. Kunin, M.D., author of *Mega-Nutrition for Women,* states that body fat must be maintained at a minimum of 18 percent for women to continue a normal menstrual cycle. Any condition that interferes with the menstrual cycle can lower bone density.

Staying Too Thin

As can exercise-induced weight loss, continual, prolonged, or on-again-off-again dieting habits can severely interfere with hormonal and calcium function. Obsession with weight and dieting leads many women to resort to extremely low calorie diets that lack sufficient amounts of calcium and other bone-building elements. This inadequate consumption, coupled with absorption problems, triggers the body to pull more calcium from bone to stabilize falling blood levels. Thin women are more at risk of osteoporosis for many reasons: they have less bone mass to start with; the body's fat stores convert androgens (hormones secreted by the adrenal glands after menopause) to estrogen, so women with less fat make less estrogen, which leads to less absorption of calcium by the bone, and this in turn leads to bone loss; and fat on bone functions in a metabolic way that causes new bone to be produced.

Supplementation

Although we should try to obtain our calcium and the other vitamins and minerals for strong healthy bones from our diets, this is becoming more and more difficult. The advent of "modern" agricultural methods has left us with a legacy of poor soil. As the quality of our soil has declined, so has the quality of our food. Minerals that were once abundant in our soil, and consequently in our food, have been depleted. Coupling this with our less-than-healthy Standard American Diet, more and more studies are reporting vast deficiencies in vitamins and minerals among Americans.

Buyer beware: not all supplements are created equal. Calcium supplements are often found as calcium compounds. The most common are calcium carbonate, calcium citrate, calcium lactate, and calcium gluconate. There have been a number of studies that have attempted to determine which form of calcium is the best absorbed. In 1987 Ralph Shangraw, Ph.D., chairman of the Department of Pharmaceutics at the University of Maryland School of Pharmacy, published the results of his analysis of 80 calcium supplements, revealing that almost half of the various brands on the market did not disintegrate and the calcium went unused. Earlier, in 1985, researchers from the University of Texas Health Sciences Center at Dallas concluded that "calcium citrate provides a more optimum calcium bioavailability than calcium carbonate." In that same year the *New England Journal of Medicine* reported on a study done by Robert Recker, M.D., of Creighton University of Omaha. Recker concluded that the calcium in citrate form was significantly better absorbed by individuals with low levels of stomach acid (common in women over 40) than was the calcium in the carbonate form.[17,18] Other absorbable forms of calcium include calcium aspartate, calcium succinate, and calcium ascorbate.

Other researchers have suggested that calcium in the form of microcrystalline hydroxyapatite (whole-bone extract) is the best absorbed calcium source. In addition studies have shown that this type of calcium not only stopped bone loss, but also regenerated bone.

While labels will list the total amount of calcium compound provided by each tablet, not every label lists the amount of *elemental calcium,* which is the amount of calcium actually available to your body. The amount of elemental calcium in each tablet depends on the form of the calcium compound used. Following is a list of the most common supplements and the percent of elemental calcium in each:

Calcium carbonate	40%
Hydroxyapatite	30%
Calcium citrate	24%
Calcium lactate	13%
Calcium gluconate	9%

For example, if the label on your supplement bottle says 1,000 mg and you are taking calcium carbonate (40 percent elemental calcium), you are actually getting only 400 mg of elemental calcium, the remaining 600 mg being carbonate. Calcium phosphate contains over 23 percent elemental calcium, but I generally do not recommend it because our diets tend to have excessive phosphorus. Bone meal (31 percent elemental calcium) and dolomite (22 percent elemental calcium) should also be avoided, since they may be contaminated with lead, toxic minerals, and pesticides.

I recommend supplementing with a product called Osteo Forte, which contains calcium in its most absorbable forms (citrate, aspartate, succinate, and ascorbate), as well as vitamin D and a whole host of trace minerals that support bone building. This supplement is available from Uni-Key Health Systems (1-800-888-4353).

When it comes to calcium, the RDA is 800 mg for ages 1 to 10; 1,200 mg, ages 11 to 18, when bone mass is being laid down; and 1,000 mg for adults. Experts at the NIH are now recommending 1,500 mg for postmenopausal women. I question the need for these high amounts. As previously mentioned, ethnic groups who have much less dietary calcium intake, such as the African Bantu, who only consume 400 mg or less of calcium a day, have a lower incidence of osteoporosis than our affluent society, where dairy calcium is an integral part of the diet. When calcium is present in balance with the other essential bone minerals, the need for calcium alone may be lowered.

Remember that food is your best source of calcium. A supplement is just that—it supplements the diet. Please refer to the list in Chapter 3 for food rich in calcium. And remember, whatever form of calcium you choose to take, you are only throwing money away if you are inhibiting the absorption of this vital mineral by continuing to drink coffee or sodas, smoke cigarettes, or avoid exercise.

Osteoporosis, perhaps more so than any other female condition, is a telltale sign of how you've been living your life over the past 20 to 30 years. It is the natural consequence of what you've been eating, how you've been exercising, your consumption of coffee and sodas, and those high-protein diets you followed from time to time. As Linda Showler, N.D., so aptly puts it in the *Townsend Letter for Doctors* (May, 1990) "What we are now witnessing is a generation of women who've been sedentary, smoked cigarettes, and consumed unprecedented quantities of protein, sugar, and coffee—all well-known risk factors for osteoporosis." Although many sources claim that absorption of calcium in the intestine typically diminishes with age, leaving us helpless against osteoporosis, I do not believe this to be inevitable, but yet another consequence of a lifetime of poor nutritional habits.

My approach to osteoporosis is like the disease itself, multifaceted. We need to be aware of *all* the factors contributing to our risk of this disease and work toward changing those factors over which we have control. We do have a choice in *how* our bodies age. We can make positive lifestyle and dietary choices that can slow down and eliminate many of the risks of developing this degenerative disease. By improving and supplementing our diets to aid in proper absorption of nutrients, by eliminating unhealthy lifestyle habits, and by participating in regular weight-bearing exercise, we can improve and support our bones. The choice is ours.

5
Heart Disease

Women's hearts, in the emotional sense, have been the subject of hundreds of thousands of volumes written by poets, novelists, and songwriters, but in comparison very little medical writing exists on the health of women's physical hearts. Yet heart attacks are the number-one killer of women in this country, with more than a quarter of a million women dying from them every year. In fact, heart attacks claim the lives of more women than all forms of cancer combined. Women who have heart attacks are twice as likely to die as their male counterparts within the first few weeks after the attack. If they survive the first year after a heart attack, women are twice as likely as men to have a second attack.

Despite these facts, almost all we know about heart disease and its treatment relates to men. Doctors, as well as female patients themselves, have classically viewed heart disease as a male problem. One reason for this is that women develop the problem about 10 years later than men do. Another reason is that women have been excluded from almost all major studies on heart disease, perhaps because the majority of doctors traditionally have been men. Those studies that *have* used women subjects have been conducted for shorter periods of time with smaller numbers of subjects and have provided less data and no long-term results. All of this leads to heart disease being ignored or undiagnosed in women, and being far more advanced by the time women seek or receive medical care. Even those who do seek care early are often not taken seriously. A 1987 study at Albert Einstein College of Medicine of Yeshiva University in New York showed that women's chest pains were more likely to be diagnosed as psychiatric than men's.

The result of all of this is that many of the diagnostic and treatment methods for heart disease that have been developed in the last couple of decades do not work as well for women as they do for men. Stress tests and even electrocardiograms (ECGs) are less accurate for women in diagnosing heart disease. Bypass surgery and angioplasty, standard treatment procedures for male patients, are less effective in their female counterparts. Although funding is now being allocated for research on women's health issues in an attempt to play catch-up, by the time many of these studies are completed, it may be the proverbial "too little, too late" for many women.

Simply put, cardiovascular disease results when the lumens of the coronary arteries, which carry blood, oxygen, and nutrients to the heart, become smaller. This constriction can be due to excess salt in the blood pulling fluid from the arteries. Arteries are further constricted by a build-up of fats, oxidized cholesterol, and plaque in the artery walls. Angina, or chest pain, occurs when the heart fails to receive enough oxygen through these narrowed arteries. When these arteries become obstructed, a heart attack can occur, resulting in damage to the heart. This process of plaque build-up and obstruction is known as atherosclerosis, or hardening of the arteries.

Hypertension, or high blood pressure, is one of the major factors contributing to cardiovascular disease, but it also occurs as a *result* of hardening of the arteries. The exact cause of hypertension is generally unknown, but what we do know is that high blood pressure often accompanies heart disease. Almost 50 percent of all midlife women are diagnosed with hypertension by age 50. Most who have hypertension are unaware of it because it usually produces no physical symptoms. Routine blood-pressure checks, at least every 2 years, can detect potential hypertension; blood pressure readings above 140/90 may spell danger.

Since so many test results have shown a direct relationship between high salt intake and hypertension, holding back the salt shaker would be wise. Sodium is a factor in hypertension because it causes fluid retention, which adds stress to both the heart and circulatory system. Hypertension, left undiagnosed or untreated, can result in stroke, heart attack, kidney failure, and other serious diseases. Over 20 percent of the adult white population and over 30 percent of the adult black population suffer from high blood pressure.

Risk Factors

Heredity plays a part in heart disease. The closer your blood tie to a relative who suffered from heart disease, the stronger your risk of developing it. Diet and lifestyle have also been clearly implicated as causative factors. Dietary factors that are related include excessive intakes of salt, sugar, and nonessential fats. An elevated serum cholesterol level is also a risk factor. Women smokers are two to six times more likely to develop heart disease than their nonsmoking counterparts. In addition, women who lead sedentary lives are also more likely to develop heart disease. These women tend to be overweight, have high blood pressure and high cholesterol levels, and many of them are also smokers. Exercise, even in moderate amounts, has been shown to increase the "good" high-density lipid (HDL) cholesterol levels, lower blood pressure, and help reduce weight. Speaking of weight, there seems to be a consensus among researchers that where you carry your fat is more important than being overweight in itself. The "apple-shaped" body (excess weight carried at the waist) seems to carry more risk of heart attack than the "pear-shaped" body (excess weight carried on the hips and thighs).

An additional female risk factor for heart disease is diabetes; blood platelets in diabetics seem to stick together more readily than in nondiabetics, causing clogging of the arteries. Research shows that women over the age of 45 are twice as likely as men to develop adult-onset diabetes, and female diabetics are at double the risk of heart disease of male diabetics. The good news is that adult-onset diabetes can be managed with diet and exercise, a subject covered more extensively in Chapter 8.

Using medication to control heart disease risk factors has negative effects. While drugs may be effective, they are designed to treat the symptoms and do nothing to change the underlying biochemical imbalances and lifestyle habits that cause the problems in the first place. In the case of high blood pressure, medications such as diuretics and beta-blockers (Inderal) are widely used. The results of several long-term studies, however, seem to indicate that these medications may actually increase the risk of heart attack. Diuretics, for example, increase the excretion of potassium and magnesium; the latter mineral has been shown effective in lowering blood pressure and preventing heart attacks. Beta-blockers work by decreasing heart rate and cardiac output, but are also known to increase cholesterol and triglyceride levels in the blood. They also have numerous side effects, including congestive heart failure. Although it may be harder to change a lifetime of bad habits, making changes in diet and exercise, and reducing weight have proved most effective in controlling and preventing heart disease.

Estrogen

Because of the lack of research specific to women and heart disease, and because women begin to show symptoms of heart disease at about the same time menopause occurs, an assumption has been made on the part of many medical researchers and practitioners that reduced levels of estrogen are a major contributing factor to heart disease in women. The result is that heart disease has been added to the list of health problems experienced by midlife women that many doctors routinely treat with estrogen replacement therapy (ERT). Yet, the results of scientific studies on estrogen and heart disease are at best contradictory and inconclusive.

While estrogen use in women seems to reduce the level of "bad" cholesterol [low-density lipids (LDL)] and increase the "good" cholesterol (HDL), it is also known to increase triglyceride levels. High triglyceride levels have been linked to increased risk of heart attack in women even when cholesterol levels are normal. Studies have also shown that estrogen has the potential to raise blood pressure and increase blood clotting. Some of the most disturbing research results were from a 60-month controlled, blind study of men who were given estrogen treatment to prevent a second heart attack; the study was stopped after 18 months due to the increase in heart attacks in the men on estrogen.[1]

While ERT seems to have become a panacea for all health problems experienced by midlife women, there are many less harmful ways of preventing heart disease than exposing women to the known and yet unknown risks of ERT. There are also more natural ways of lowering blood pressure and reducing the risk of heart attack than using diuretics, beta-blockers, and cholesterol-lowering drugs. No matter how old we are, we need to take control of our own body and give it the optimum nutrition needed to naturally protect against hypertension and heart disease.

Magnesium and the Heart

Just as the role of magnesium, boron, and the other essential vitamins and trace minerals in osteoporosis has been overshadowed by the focus on calcium, the role of magnesium in heart disease has been virtually ignored due to the cholesterol craze and emphasis on estrogen. We all know that high cholesterol levels are somehow related to heart disease, but most of us are unaware that magnesium deficiencies can result in such heart conditions as irregular heartbeat, rapid heartbeat, high blood pressure, and sudden death. Magnesium deficiencies may also be the cause of idiopathic mitral valve prolapse, a heart valve disorder whose symptoms include palpitations, chest pain, fatigue, panic attacks, and hyperventilation. This common disorder affects about 5 percent of the population. Low levels of both blood and cellular magnesium have been reported in individuals with high blood pressure and hypertension, and biopsies reveal that individuals who die from heart attacks have lower magnesium levels in their heart muscle.

To add to the problem, the diuretics or fluid pills often prescribed to treat the swelling and fluid retention caused by high blood pressure *cause* both magnesium and potassium deficiencies. The powerful cardiac drug digitalis also affects both magnesium and potassium utilization. Often, potassium is prescribed along with digitalis, and magnesium is neglected. This is unsound nutritional medicine, because the body requires magnesium in order to use potassium. Therefore, a primary magnesium deficiency is tantamount to a potassium deficiency. Drugs that are used to treat dysrhythmia (irregular heart beat), such as quinidine sulfate and disopyramide phosphate, are also known to induce a magnesium deficiency. Magnesium supplementation, in addition to the generally prescribed potassium, should be part of every nutritional protocol for women taking cardiac drugs.

Magnesium deficiencies can actually hasten the development of atherosclerosis, or hardening of the arteries. If calcium is not kept in balance with magnesium, it is unable to become part of the bone. This unused calcium then gets dumped into the arteries and becomes part of the "hardened" artery. With the current pumping of supplemental calcium into every possible food and beverage, excess calcium, out of balance with magnesium and other minerals, is surely floating around in many of our arteries. Bringing magnesium levels back into balance with calcium can deter the accumulation of calcium in the blood vessels.

Instead of assessing magnesium levels and increasing this important mineral to its proper ratio with calcium, the doctors of many heart patients with potential magnesium deficiencies are prescribing *calcium channel blockers*. These include Procardia, Cardizem, Cardene, Cardalate, and Isoptin or Calan, and are being used to prevent heart muscle spasms by blocking excess calcium from being absorbed into the heart muscle. Magnesium is a natural calcium channel blocker; it dilates coronary arteries and peripheral arteries when available in sufficient levels and in balance with calcium, yet it is overlooked as a key factor in maintaining a healthy heart.

As important as magnesium's role in bone health and osteoporosis, it is vital to muscle health and in the prevention and treatment of heart disease. While calcium is needed to make muscles contract, magnesium is need for them to relax, and where the heart is concerned, this is crucial because if the heart is under constant stress, it cannot function properly. Numerous studies have linked hard drinking water, high in magnesium and calcium content, with low rates of serious heart disease. In fact, intravenous magnesium has been successfully used for over 50 years in the treatment of coronary spasms and heart attacks.[2]

Sufficient magnesium also has been shown to lower total cholesterol, LDL cholesterol, and triglyceride levels while raising HDL cholesterol.[3] This is especially good news for women because diets designed to lower LDL levels often lower HDL levels as well, which in women leads to an increase risk of heart disease. In addition, magnesium has been found to reduce platelet aggregation, the stickiness of blood cells that contributes to their clumping in the arteries.

A USDA nationwide food consumption survey found that the typical American diet provides only one-half to two-thirds of the recommended 400 mg of magnesium a day. Some experts recommend up to 800 to 1,000 mg of magnesium. The depletion of our soil and the overprocessing and overcooking of our food robs it of much of its magnesium content. Excesses in sugar, alcohol, fiber, caffeine, "bad" fats, and phosphates in sodas and other processed foods sap our bodies of magnesium, as does that ever-present twentieth-century condition: stress. Table 5-1 (pages 98–99) lists foods that are high in magnesium.

The traditional blood test to measure magnesium is considered useless in assessing magnesium deficiency, because the body tries to maintain a balance of magnesium in the blood at all times. When blood levels drop, magnesium is pulled from other parts of the body, so blood tests generally show adequate levels of magnesium, when in reality the individual may be severely deficient. One of the most accurate diagnostic tests available at the present is called the magnesium loading test, which tests the urine rather than the blood. You might want to ask your doctor about it.

Cholesterol: Maligned and Misunderstood

Almost all of us have been made aware of the basic theory of cholesterol and heart disease. We know that

Table 5-1
Foods High in Magnesium

Food	Mg/100 g Edible Portion*
Kelp	760
Wheat bran	490
Wheat germ	336
Almonds	270
Cashews	267
Blackstrap molasses	258
Brewer's yeast	231
Buckwheat	229
Brazil nut	225
Dulse	220
Filberts	184
Peanuts	175
Millet	162
Wheat grain	160
Pecan	142
English walnut	131
Rye	115
Tofu	111
Coconut meat, dry	90
Soybeans, cooked	88
Spinach (raw)	88
Brown rice	88
Dried figs	71
Swiss chard	65
Apricots, dried (unsulphured)	62
Dates	58
Collard leaves	57
Shrimp	51
Sweet corn	48

Food	Mg/100 g Edible Portion*
Avocado	45
Cheddar cheese	45
Parsley	41
Prunes, dried	40

*100 g = 3.5 oz.
(Data from Endo-met Laboratories, Phoenix, AZ, based on evaluation of existing literature.)

cholesterol is carried through the bloodstream in two protein factions, HDL and LDL. The HDL is considered the "good" cholesterol, and the LDL the "bad." An excess of LDL increases our risk of heart attacks or strokes, while high levels of HDL are protective. In general, total cholesterol levels higher than 200 can be a sign of increased risk for heart disease. In women, LDL levels should be below 130 and optimum HDL levels should be greater than 65. More important than just these single levels, the ratio of total cholesterol to HDL should be below 4:1.

What many of us are not aware of is the fact that cholesterol is found naturally in every cell in our body and that each cell also contains enzymes used for the production of cholesterol. Our brains and spinal cord contain about 25 percent of the cholesterol in our bodies. This important substance is found in the skin, where it is converted to vitamin D by sunlight; in the marrow of our bones, where blood cells are formed; and in our adrenal glands, where it is used in the formation of sex hormones, especially those found in postmenopausal women. Cholesterol is essential to good health, and deficiencies have been associated with anemia, acute infection, and excess thyroid function. In our diets, cholesterol is the waxy fatlike substances found only in products of animal origin, such as beef, poultry, and eggs.

So, if cholesterol is so vitally important to our health, why have we been led to believe we need to avoid it in our diets? The concern over cholesterol in our diets began with a 1913 Russian study by Nikolai Anitschkov, a physiologist. He found that feeding rabbits huge doses of cholesterol caused a dramatic rise in cholesterol in their blood. The resulting hardening of the arteries was blamed on cholesterol because it was found at the site of arterial damage. From this, the theory developed that diets high in cholesterol caused heart disease, and an advertising campaign was launched promoting the idea that processed substitutes for dairy items, eggs, and butter are healthier for us than the natural foods on which they are based.

Yet the relationship between high levels of dietary cholesterol and high levels of blood cholesterol may surprise you. Studies from the University of California, Los Angeles, the University of Missouri, and others find no correlation between cholesterol in the diet and heart attack rates. Neither the Pritikin low-fat diet nor the American Heart Association limited-fat diet lowered blood cholesterol levels in patients with early vascular disease in a year-long Canadian study. In a 1965 British study, patients who had had a heart attack were placed on either a low-fat diet supplemented with 4 tbsp. of corn oil per day, or a diet high in saturated fats and cholesterol. Even though serum cholesterol levels fell in the corn-oil diet group, they had nearly twice as many heart attacks as the saturated-fat diet group. Results from two separate studies involving the use of cholesterol-lowering drugs have baffled researchers: although cholesterol levels were lowered and deaths from heart-related problems were significantly less in the groups taking the drug, deaths from violent causes, including suicides, homicides, and accidents, increased threefold.

What this research seems to suggest is the amount of cholesterol in one's blood *is* related to heart disease, while the amount of cholesterol in one's diet *is not. What does lead to high blood cholesterol is the lack of other nutrients—such as chromium, magnesium, vitamin B₃, and omega-3 essential fatty acids—to metabolize it.* In addition, recent research findings have documented that cholesterol accumulates in arteries only *after* the arterial wall has been damaged. Cholesterol, in and of itself, is not the villain it has been made out to be.

Pure, fresh cholesterol does not damage arteries, but oxygenated cholesterol does. Cholesterol that has been exposed to oxygen produces toxic substances that decompose into *free radicals,* a term that has become synonymous with cell and tissue destruction. Re-examination of the Anitschkov and other animal feeding studies have found that the cholesterol used was not in the form that it occurs naturally in food, but was crystalline cholesterol in the form of heat-dried egg-yolk powder made up in batches to last many days or weeks. This altered cholesterol, because of its exposure to oxygen, formed free radicals.

Free radicals are present in cholesterol that has oxidized due to exposure to air, high temperatures, free radical initiators, light, or a combination of all these factors. Free radicals are unstable and highly reactive oxygen molecules with unpaired electrons. They search for and steal an electron from other molecules, causing a chemical reaction that creates even more free radicals. It is free radicals that cause the damage to our blood vessel walls. They also cause other damage within cells by attacking membranes, proteins, and DNA.

According to a 1979 study by C. B. Taylor, M.D., oxidized cholesterol from food sources that are left out at room temperature or are fried, smoked, cured (sausage), or aged (cheese) can be highly atherogenic (plaque-producing).[4] Cholesterol in our diets is dangerous only when it becomes oxidized, and processing, packaging, storage, and preparing of foods has a profound effect on oxidation. Foods that cause problems because of their chemically altered cholesterol are any animal food that has been exposed to ravages of oxygen for extended periods of time, for example, improperly stored eggs, milk, or butter that is exposed to room temperature for long periods of time or not stored in tightly sealed containers. Other sources of oxidized cholesterol can be found in many "fast foods"—fried chicken, fish, and hamburgers. Dried milk, dried eggs, and packaged dry baking mixes (for custards, cakes, puddings, pancakes) are also on the list. Some of the greatest sources of oxidized cholesterol include dried and powdered egg and milk products, and packaged dry baking mixes, the very products being touted and recommended for their cholesterol-lowering effects!

All of this is not to say that diets high in fats and cholesterol are not related to heart disease, but the relationship is different than we have been led to believe. Fats and cholesterol don't just clog up arteries. They *are* a major source of those nasty molecules, the free radicals, which oxidize cells and set off a chain reaction, creating more and more free radicals.

To make matters worse, the cholesterol manufactured by our bodies to fight against the damage done by free radicals is converted into its oxidized form. This only leads to more free radicals.

So how do we stop this chain reaction? We need to prevent the oxidation of cholesterol. By avoiding foods that contain oxidized cholesterol and damaged fats, and increasing our intake of foods rich in antioxidant vitamins, minerals, and essential fatty acids (EFAs), women can decrease their risk of heart disease. Antioxidants are nutrients capable of neutralizing free radicals. These nutrients are not produced by our bodies, but need to come from diet and supplementation. More and more research is indicating that heart disease is related to deficiencies of these nutrients, including vitamins E, C, and A and the minerals selenium, chromium, zinc, and magnesium.

Heart-healthy diets, low in fat and cholesterol and designed to lower serum cholesterol levels, are a standard recommendation for anyone with elevated cholesterol. While these diets have proven effective for men, they may spell trouble for women. For women, levels of "good" HDL cholesterol are key. HDL levels above 65 are now considered the most desirable; levels between 45 and 65 indicate borderline risk of heart disease. "Bad" LDL cholesterol levels should optimally be less than 130. Levels between 130 and 159 suggest borderline risk, while levels greater than 159 indicate high risk. Some special diets, such as one endorsed by the American Heart Association, reduce LDL levels in men without affecting HDL levels. But, in women, this same diet results in reduction of both LDL and HDL. In men, the risk of heart disease seems to be primarily affected by a rise in LDL levels. In women, however, lowering HDL levels may increase their risk of heart disease even if LDL levels are lowered at the same time. Luckily there are a number of easy-to-take nutrients that can help us. Both chromium and vitamin C have been shown to lower plasma cholesterol while increasing HDL levels.[5-7] Chromium is well known for its role in cholesterol metabolism and protects the lining of the arteries from damage, thereby preventing build-up of cholesterol in the arteries.

Ishwarial Jialal, M.D., at the University of Texas Southwestern Medical Center has shown that vitamin C is 95 percent effective in inhibiting LDL oxidation in a test tube. Beta carotene was 90 percent effective and vitamin E, 45 percent. K. Fred Gey, M.D., and his colleagues at the Institute of Biochemistry and Molecular Biology in Bern, Switzerland, found that low blood levels of vitamin E are a better predictor of heart disease than cholesterol levels or blood pressure. Vitamin E has long been known as a potent antioxidant. It has been shown to scavenge free radicals and increase internal antioxidation. Vitamin E also helps thin the blood. It inhibits blood platelets from becoming sticky, thereby reducing blood clotting problems. This is especially beneficial for women, who do not seem to be able to tolerate the one-a-day blood thinning aspirin routine. Vitamin E is also protective of two other antioxidant vitamins, A and C. When E is present, less A and C is required.

Fiber in the form of oat bran and psyllium husks has proved effective in lowering LDL and raising HDL, and used in tasty oat bran muffins and cleansing drinks. The old standbys, garlic and olive oil, are other foods that seem to be beneficial to women's cholesterol levels. The omega-3 fatty acids found in fish oils, fish, and vegetable oils such as flax are heart smart because they dramatically reduce both cholesterol and triglycerides without affecting the beneficial HDLs. Another attractive benefit is their ability to lower blood pressure. Flax oil is a buttery, nutty-tasting oil that makes a good butter substitute. It can be drizzled over steamed vegetables, cooked cereals, and air-popped popcorn for a rich, satisfying flavor. Flax oil should not be used for cooking as heat destroys its value.

Fat

It is interesting to note that within the past 100 years there has been a 350 percent increase in cardio-vascular disease, but the cholesterol content of the American diet has remained about the same. During this same 100 years, however, both sugar and processed oil consumption has risen considerably. Hydrogenated polyunsaturated oils, including margarine, have been recommended for years in cholesterol-lowering diets. And while it is true that they will reduce cholesterol levels, it is also true that they accelerate arteriosclerosis and other degenerative disease. Why? Because oils that have been commercially processed to improve shelf life, flavor, smell, and color have been damaged. In the processing, high temperatures convert the polyunsaturated fatty acids from the naturally occurring beneficial "cis" to the unnatural, harmful "trans" form. Cis fats melt at 55 degrees, well below the normal body temperature of 98.6°F, which makes them fully available to the system. Trans fats melt at up to 111°F, so they remain solid, and therefore unmetabolized, in the human body.

The process of hydrogenation, which converts liquid oils into hardened fats such as margarine and vegetable shortening, destroys natural fatty acids in even greater numbers, converting them into the biologically impaired trans form. Trans fats, found in all processed oils on your grocery shelves and in margarines (which have the highest percentage of trans fatty acids), cannot be used by the body to produce prostaglandins, hormone-like compounds that regulate every function in the human body at the molecular level. These trans fats interfere with normal cell membrane function and structure, and block the good healthy fats, such as raw natural oils that make prostaglandins, from being taken in. In addition to these trans fats, the hydrogenation process also removes the very nutrients that are essential for healthy hearts—vitamins E and B_6, chromium, and magnesium.

Triglycerides

Although triglycerides are another type of blood fat, they are covered here separately because of their relationship in women to heart disease. As stated earlier, high triglyceride levels in women are known to increase susceptibility to heart disease even when cholesterol levels are normal. Many experts say that triglyceride levels above 190 are cause for concern; I believe that triglyceride levels above 100 are cause for concern. In our diets we take in triglycerides in the form of fats and oils, and our livers manufacture it from refined sugars. In our bloodstreams, sticky triglyceride particles function like glue, causing red corpuscles to clump and stick together. This results in the blockage of small capillaries, leading to oxygen starvation of the tissues and organs served by these capillaries. Triglycerides are also the form in which the body stores fat in the connective tissue. The roll above many a middle-aged stomach is actually excess triglycerides.

What we eat and the way we live affect our triglyceride levels. Too much refined carbohydrates, typical of the American diet, accounts for elevated triglyceride levels. White sugar, white flour, and products such as white bread, cakes, cookies, candies, soda, and alcohol all increase our triglyceride levels. Even too much fruit and natural, unsweetened fruit juice can result in elevated levels. Although ingestion of fat alone can double triglyceride levels, coupling fat ingestion with alcohol consumption increases the levels three and a half times. A few drinks before a fatty meal that is followed by a sugary desert can spell disaster.

Not only what we eat, but the *way* we eat affects our triglyceride levels. By skipping breakfast and/or lunch and making up for it with our evening meal, a diet pattern many women fall into, blood triglycerides are increased. Eating a large meal late in the day is like putting gas in your car and then leaving it parked in the garage; the fuel is not used. In the body, unused triglycerides are stored in fatty tissue; skipping breakfast the next day results in those triglycerides flooding out of the fatty tissue and sludging up the bloodstream. Our bodies were designed to be fueled at regular intervals with good balanced food. If we're not eating regularly, we're damaging our bodies.

Other contributing factors to high triglyceride levels over which we have control include lack of physical activity; our reaction to emotional stress; and consumption of caffeine, nicotine, certain drugs such as diuretics and birth control pills, and some hormones, including estrogen. Since both triglyceride and cholesterol levels increase naturally with age, we should have them checked every couple of years as a routine part of our health care.

The Supernutrition Dietary Overview

Hold That Salt

Keeping tabs on the sodium content of our foods is a must to help prevent high blood pressure and stroke. The first step is to remove most processed foods from the diet because they are the highest sources of sodium. This means limiting or eliminating most canned, pickled, smoked, instant and snack foods from the diet. Also note that dairy products are high in sodium (unless unsalted). Become a label reader and avoid anything than contains the word *sodium* on the label, such as monosodium glutamate, sodium benzoate, sodium nitrate, and disodium phosphate. Even baking soda and baking powder are sodium-rich. Try to keep your daily sodium intake down to 2,000 mg. Remember that 1 tsp. of salt equals 2,000 mg of sodium; 1 tbsp. of soy sauce contains 1,029 mg of sodium.

Heart-Smart Oils

As we have seen, the wrong fat can be devastating for us. The right fat, however, can be healing. EFAs not only help prevent heart disease, they are vital for overall good health. Flax seed, sesame, olive, and canola are the oils of choice in the Prime-Time Diet. These oils provide us with essential and healthy fats as well as heart-protecting nutrients, such as lecithin, beta carotene, and vitamin E, that have been removed from processed oils.

Flax seed oil is the best vegetable source of omega-3s, the type of fat that lowers triglyceride and bad cholesterol levels and is most deficient in today's American diet. Flax seed oil's incredible oxygen-absorbing ability helps to oxygenate the body. (This positive feature should not be confused with the negative effects of oxidized cholesterol.) Due to its high polyunsaturate chemical profile, it is very sensitive to light, heat, and air. It is best used in no-heat recipes, drizzled on cooked vegetables, or as a butter substitute in hot cereals. It has a nutty, rich flavor that may take some getting used to.

Sesame oil gets rave reviews because of its mild nutty flavor and high versatility. It contains sesamol, a natural antioxidant that makes it very stable and highly resistant to oxidation. It also has a fairly high monounsaturated fat content, making it a good heart protector. This oil is good for sautéing, baking, and as a salad dressing.

Most of us are familiar with the virtues of olive oil, a full-bodied oil used almost to the exclusion of other oils in the Mediterranean region, where heart disease and cancer rates are much lower than ours. Olive oil is a monounsaturated oil, which means it is very stable against the free radical effects of heat, air, and light. "Extra virgin" olive oil is a wonderful oil for both cooking and using on salads. It is a highly beneficial oil for women because it has been shown to reduce LDL levels while keeping HDL levels high.

Canola oil has a fatty acid profile similar to olive oil. It was developed by the Canadians, hence the word *can*ola and is derived from the rapeseed plant. Canola is the oil lowest in saturated fat and, like flax seed oil, contains beneficial omega-3s. Its mild taste makes it an ideal choice for those who do not want the rich taste of olive oil in their cooking. Its high smoking point is another reason why it is one of the best oils for cooking. There is now a new "margarine substitute" on the market made from canola oil. The product, known as Spectrum Spread, is available in health food stores.

When purchasing oils, look for the words *expeller pressed* and *organic*. Name brands to look for include Spectrum Naturals, Arrowhead Mills, Erewhon, and Flora. These oils will be more expensive, but their good health dividends are priceless.

Besides these protective oils, foods rich in the antioxidant nutrients vitamins A, C, and E, beta carotene, and selenium are a must for healthy hearts. Fresh fruits, leafy green vegetables, a variety of whole grains, freshly squeezed vegetable juices, sea vegetables, garlic, and onions are good sources of these important nutrients. In addition, garlic, combined with cayenne pepper, is one of the best combinations for lowering blood pressure naturally. Fiber, particularly the soluble fiber found in fruits, vegetables, barley, and oats, helps to lower cholesterol levels, and assists in eliminating toxins and carcinogens from the digestive tract.

Foods to avoid include all commercially processed oils, whole-milk dairy products, sugar, white flour, fried foods, hydrogenated fats such as margarine and vegetable shortenings, and soybean oil. It would also be wise to limit our intake of red meat, regular salt, coffee, and alcohol.

6
Other Midlife Concerns:

Breast Cancer, Diabetes, and Hypothyroidism

The Supernutrition Approach to Breast Cancer

As a practicing nutritionist dealing with women's issues, I have become keenly aware over the years that women are terrified more of breast cancer than of any other disease. While breast cancer rates are increasing —up a staggering 60 percent since 1950—more women are surviving the disease, probably due to earlier detection. But the treatment is what women fear most: disfiguring surgery and, in many cases, months of debilitating chemotherapy and radiation therapy. Because the treatment choices for this dreaded disease are so physically and emotionally devastating, prevention is even more fundamentally important than early detection.

Both heredity and lifestyle factors play strong roles in the incidence of breast cancer. Researchers almost universally agree that breast cancer in women before menopause is more connected to heredity, while occurrence after menopause is more the result of lifestyle influences such as diet and environment. Breast cancer is more common in Western cultures and strikes white women more often than women of color. It occurs in women more often after the age of 50, and more frequently in women who are obese. Smoking has also been tied to breast cancer. In addition, the following five characteristics have been identified by researchers as common in women who develop breast cancer; this does not necessarily mean that if you fit one or more of these characteristics that you will get breast cancer, but the risk is there:

- A mother or sister who has had breast cancer
- Having had cancer in one breast
- Never having borne a child and being past the age to do so
- Being over 30 at the time of your first pregnancy
- Beginning menstruation early (before the age of 12, or entering menopause late (after the age of 55)

One factor that comes into play after menopause over which we have control is long-term estrogen replacement therapy. Most commonly prescribed to prevent osteoporosis and heart disease, ERT alone has been found to increase the chances of developing uterine cancer five to seven times. With breast cancer, however, the picture is not as clear. As I researched the topic, I learned that there have been close to 2,000 studies on the estrogen–breast connection. Some studies suggested that ERT increased the risk for breast cancer, others concluded it did not, and some implicated it only with long-term use (10 years or more). Needless to say, I was confused. I was relieved to come across the result of a review by researchers from the Center for Disease Prevention and Health Promotion in Atlanta.[1] These researchers reviewed all valid epidemiological studies on estrogen and breast cancer. In studies that met the highest standards for research methods employed, ERT was consistently shown to increase the risk of breast cancer by 4 percent per year. When multiplied by 15 years, the length of time some women will remain on ERT, the risk is a whopping 60 percent! I believe these results speak for themselves.

It is even more disconcerting to consider that the latest research studies from Sweden and the University of Southern California conclude that when progesterone is added to estrogen replacement therapy, the risk of breast cancer is doubled after 10 years.

There are two diagnostic tests that can help women detect any abnormalities in the breast before full-blown breast cancer develops. The first is breast self-examination. The American Cancer Society suggests that women practice breast examination about a week after the end of their menstrual period. For those past menopause, examine the first day of each month. Your doctor's office or your local American Cancer Society chapter can provide you with information on how to do your own breast examination. A second early detection method is mammograms. These breast x-rays can spotlight small growths that cannot be found through self-examination. The American Cancer Society recommends a baseline mammogram at age 35. A mammogram is recommended every 2 years after age 40; after age 50, every year. Remember to include supplemental antioxidants—particularly extra vitamin C, vitamin A and selenium the day before, the day of and the day after a mammogram to protect against free radicals from x-ray exposure.

Lifestyle habits that contribute to your risk are things you can control. What you eat, what you drink, and what you weigh are important. According to the American Cancer Society, overweight women have a 55 percent higher chance of dying from cancer than those of normal weight. And while high dietary fat intake has become the focus of breast cancer risk, the role of sugar has been ignored. In truth, both animal and human research studies have connected breast cancer with high-sugar diets. Since our country has become so fat-phobic, sugar consumption has skyrocketed to a startling 120 pounds per person, per year. Along with this rise in sugar consumption, there has been a rise in breast cancer rates. A landmark study correlating data from no fewer than 21 countries revealed that sugar presents a major risk, for women over 45, of the development of breast cancer.[2] Given the relationship between excess sugar and calcium loss from the body, it would seem that getting sugar out of the diet as much as we can should be a primary focus for women's health.

As many of us already know, high-fat diets have also been implicated in breast cancer. After carefully reviewing the studies, it is my opinion that it may be more a question of the kind of fat consumed rather than the amounts. I base this statement on the fact that women in Mediterranean countries show a low level of breast cancer yet consume a high-fat diet (40 percent of total calories); the key seems to be that the fat they consume is monounsaturated olive oil. Animal studies have confirmed that when test animals are fed olive oil–rich diets they show fewer breast tumors than animals on a high–polyunsaturated fat diet. Japanese women, eating their native diets, consume fat in the form of cold-water fish, a rich source of omega-3 fatty acids. Their breast cancer rates are four times less than American women. Once these Japanese start eating a Western diet, which includes different kinds of fat, they begin to show cancer rates nearer the higher American levels. Greenland Eskimos, whose diets are uncommonly high in fat (also in the form of fish oils), rarely develop breast cancer.

The USDA food studies of the 1980s confirm that, due to cholesterol and fat worries, women have dramatically reduced their consumption of artery-clogging saturated fats from whole milk, red meat, and eggs. However, even though we seem to be reducing fat intake, the truth is that women have merely shifted their source of fat from saturated to commercially processed polyunsaturated fat or hydrogenated fat found in corn, safflower, soybean oil or margarine, which are touted by advertisers to lower cholesterol. Total dietary fat is still at a too-high level of 37 percent of total calories, and breast cancer rates are still on the rise with 1 in 9 women developing breast cancer.

The seemingly healthful polyunsaturated substitutes may actually be worse for the female breast. Laboratory tests have shown that breast tumors appeared more frequently in animals fed diets high in safflower and corn oil than in those fed olive oil. In addition, researchers have noted dramatically higher levels of toxic chemicals such as dichlorodphenyltrichloroethane (DDT), and polychlorinated biphenyls (PCBs) in women with breast cancer. So again, it may not be simply the fat in the diet but what is in the fat.

Toxic environmental wastes are stored in fatty tissue, and the breast is a primary fatty tissue in women. This means organically grown food is your best bet.

Researchers have also observed an association between accumulated waste materials in the intestinal tract and toxic accumulations in women's breasts. The buildup of waste in the intestinal tract is due in large part to a diet lacking in fiber. Fiber is the non-nutritive element in plant foods that is indigestible to the human body. It speeds the time it takes food to pass through the intestinal tract so that noxious wastes are removed from the system quickly. Food that remains in the intestinal tract too long can ferment and putrefy, producing toxic chemicals that are released into the bloodstream. In women these wastes can eventually get dumped in breast tissue. The build-up of waste materials in the intestine can result from simple constipation; an association between constipation and breast cancer has also been seen. Therefore, increasing fiber in your diet to keep your system "swept out" helps to prevent the accumulation of toxic wastes in the intestine as well as in the breast tissue.

In the 1960s, British doctors who studied African populations discovered a strong relationship between high fiber intake and a low rate of degenerative diseases. Due to the enormous amount of refined and processed foods we consume, the average American diet contains only between 8 and 11 g of fiber; the recommended daily requirement is between 20 and 30 g. Lack of dietary fiber has been linked to a whole host of diseases common in Western society, such as heart disease, diabetes, high blood pressure, hemorrhoids, varicose veins, food allergies, and various cancers, including breast cancer.

Painful lumps in the breasts, known as fibrocystic breast disease or benign breast disease, affect 60 percent of all women during their lives. Although not considered a risk factor for breast cancer, it creates fear in women nevertheless. Since cystic breasts can make self-examination difficult, a mammogram may be the best way to go for women with this condition. Diets high in caffeine and the related chemical methylxanthine from coffee, sodas, chocolate, cocoa, and tea have been strongly connected to fibrocystic breast disease. I have found that when caffeine and caffeine-related foods, even decaffeinated coffee, were *totally* removed from the diet, painful breast lumps disappeared. Breast lumps have been found to be dramatically reduced by the intake of 600 IU of vitamin E daily. The topical use of natural progesterone cream also reduces breast cysts.

Heart-Healthy Oils

Flax seed, sesame, olive, and canola are some of the best oils for overall health, including breast cancer prevention. I was fascinated to learn that in Germany, Johanna Budwig, M.D., has documented the anticancer properties of flax oil in her treatment of over 1,000 patients, including women with breast cancer. The United States is finally catching up to what the Europeans have known for a long time; the National Cancer Institute has chosen flax oil, the vegetable source with the highest levels of the beneficial omega-3 fatty acid, as a designer food for the 1990s because of its promise in preventing breast cancer. I specifically recommend at least 1 tbsp. of flax oil a day, used in its unheated form. The other oils can be used in cooking in amounts of up to 2 tbsp. a day.

Cut back on foods high in nonessential and hydrogenated fat such as pork, full-fat dairy products, margarines, vegetable shortenings, and processed vegetable oils. Increase fiber-rich whole grains, fruits and vegetables; eat five servings a day of a variety of fruits and vegetables. Eat fruits and vegetables in their whole form rather than juice and leave the peels on as much as possible, as the skins contain fiber and other nutrients.

You might want to emphasize certain vegetables in your diet. The cruciferous vegetables, including broccoli, bok choy, cauliflower, Brussels sprouts, and cabbage, are rich sources of a nitrogen-like compound called indole. (Cabbage should be *cooked* because in the raw stage a natural occurring compound called thiouracil blocks thyroid function.) The indole compound is believed to help deactivate excess estrogen in the body (which fuels cancer). Beta carotene–rich foods also appear to be powerful cancer fighters. Carrots, squash, sweet potatoes, yams, cantaloupes, peaches, and dark green leafy vegetables such as kale, collard, spinach, and mustard greens all contain healthy amounts of beta carotene. Soybeans are the newest addition to the list of protectors against cancer. Soybeans contain phyto-estrogen, a plant-based estrogen that keeps estrogen in check, thereby helping to control abnormal cell growth. You may want to experiment with a few soy-based dishes such as tempeh or tofu once or twice a week.

Garlic is an age-old, time-honored remedy, used for centuries for myriad health problems. It is only recently that science has begun to pay the respect due this "stinking rose." A whole host of research studies show garlic to be beneficial in lowering cholesterol, controlling infection, boosting immunity, protecting the body from environmental pollution, and lowering blood sugar, as well as preventing cancer. Specific to breast cancer, aged garlic extracts have been shown to inhibit the growth of breast cancer cells in the test tube. Garlic, incorporated in cooking or taken as a prepared extract, just may give us an easy ounce of prevention for breast cancer.

Do avoid all meat and poultry products that have been deliberately fed or implanted with synthetic hormones to speed their growth. Synthetic hormones such as diethylstibesterol (DES) are forms of estrogen. Residues remain in the meat, and eating large quantities assures a hefty dose of secondhand drugs. Residues, as I have mentioned, have a tendency to be stored in fatty tissues, especially the breasts. Look for hormone- and antibiotic-free meat and poultry from organic producers. Many of my clients have reported more energy when they eat organically grown lean red meat once or twice a week. Organically grown poultry products can be consumed more frequently.

Diabetes

Diabetes, often called the "woman's disease," strikes twice as many women as men over the age of 45. In fact, diabetes is one of most common diseases facing women as we grow older. The exact reason for this is unknown. We do know that obesity, whether in males or females, is perhaps the most significant factor in adult-onset diabetes. Researchers suggest that multiple pregnancies in women may be one contributing factor. Another factor in diabetes etiology is lack of strenuous physical exercise.

There are actually two types of diabetes: juvenile and adult-onset. Heredity plays a strong role in both.

Juvenile diabetes generally develops quite suddenly during childhood, and in many cases is triggered by a virus. It progresses swiftly to the point where little or no insulin is produced by the pancreas, and insulin must be taken by injection. Adult-onset diabetes does not generally develop until age 35 or later. It is less severe than the juvenile type, with insulin being deficient rather than totally lacking. This type of diabetes develops most commonly in overweight individuals, the elderly, and the poor, probably because of poor dietary choices emphasizing fats, sweets, and sugary foods. In fact, a diet high in both fats and sweets can lead to diabetes in an otherwise healthy person. The adult diabetic has some ability to produce insulin and so the condition can usually be kept under control through weight loss, diet, exercise, or oral hypoglycemic pills. The major symptoms of adult-onset diabetes include constant thirst, frequent urination at night, excessive fatigue, poor circulation, and unexplained weight loss.

Diabetes can be medically diagnosed by a fasting blood test that measures blood sugar levels. When the glucose reading is greater than 130 mg per 100 ml, a positive diagnosis can be made. Borderline diabetics have glucose levels ranging from 100 to 130 mg per ml of blood. It is a good idea to have this test done on two separate occasions.

In a healthy individual, after food is ingested the pancreas secretes the hormone insulin to regulate glucose (blood sugar) metabolism in all body tissues, especially the liver, muscle, and stored body fat. In the adult-onset diabetic, the cells that secrete insulin become degenerated or suppressed and blood sugar levels remain high. The excess glucose in the blood has many damaging effects on the kidneys, the arteries, the eyes, and the nerves. Obesity is connected to this process in two ways: (1) in obese individuals, the insulin-secreting cells are not as responsive to blood glucose levels for some unknown reason, and (2) the number of insulin receptors in special target cells are markedly decreased. So, weight loss alone can sometimes control or cure adult-onset diabetes. Exercise can also burn blood sugar like insulin and so has an important role in the diabetic's lifestyle.

The Super Nutrition Approach to Diabetes

Regulating our sugar is crucial in the prevention and control of diabetes. We need to eliminate all products that are high in sugar and white flour, such as cookies, cakes, pies, ice cream, candy, and pastries. Even concentrated carbohydrates from natural sources such as honey and fruit juices are a constant challenge to the pancreas. In addition to these foods, excessive nonessential fats that women tend to eat, especially those found in full-fat dairy products such as butter, cheese, and ice cream, block insulin activity in the blood.

Fiber is the key element in the diet to combat diabetes. Processed and refined carbohydrates should be limited. Instead we need to emphasize more complex carbohydrates from vegetables, fruits, beans, and whole grains, which provide greater fiber to help slow the release of sugar into the bloodstream. Three or more servings per day of fiber-rich foods are suggested. When increasing our fiber intake, we also need to increase our water intake to help move the fiber through the intestines. If you don't drink enough liquid, fiber can cause constipation.

A good way to reduce the craving for sweets is to keep protein levels steady. For this reason, I suggest you include at least two 3-oz. servings of fish, poultry, and other foods high in protein (lowfat cheese, beans, tempeh) each day, including up to 4 eggs per week. Lean red meat (hormone free) can be consumed once or twice a week. Refer to Chapter 8 for the complete food plan, menus, and shopping lists. You might also consider adding herbs such as cedar berries and blueberry leaf (as a tea) to your diet. These herbs have been used for centuries by herbalists to aid in the control of diabetes. Cinnamon, about one-quarter teaspoon a day, can also help diabetics by keeping glucose levels steady. Research at the U.S.D.A.'s Human Nutrition Research Center has shown that cinnamon helps insulin to metabolize blood sugar with nine times greater efficiency.

Two specific minerals, zinc and chromium, act as insulin cofactors and should be supplements to the diabetic's diet. Zinc forms part of the insulin component secreted by the pancreas and is directly involved in the body's metabolism of carbohydrates; it also has a powerful influence on wound healing and disease resistance, two factors important for diabetics, who can suffer from impaired healing and lowered immunity. Some of the best sources of zinc are lean red meats, eggs, pumpkin seeds, whole-grain cereals, and dried beans and legumes. A supplement containing 25 mg of zinc should be considered if you are not fond of these foods.

Chromium, an essential trace mineral, is absolutely necessary for proper insulin function because it regulates the metabolism of sugar. This mineral is useful for both diabetics and hypoglycemics, those with low blood sugar. In animal studies, chromium deficiency was shown to cause diabetes and was reversed with the addition of chromium. In human diabetics, ingestion of chromium resulted in the normalization of glucose tolerance tests in 50 percent of the patients tested. New studies suggest chromium helps control hunger, burns calories, and in athletes increases endurance and assists in gaining muscle and losing fat. A recent survey done by the USDA found that 9 out of 10 Americans were deficient in this critical mineral. Once again, food processing and chromium-depleted soils leave little of this mineral available to us through food. The best food sources seem to be brewer's yeast and wheat germ. I suggest dietary supplements (at least 200 mcg once or twice a day with meals) to assure adequate levels because most people don't eat enough chromium-rich foods.

There is good news for those diabetics who don't always eat properly. The Sansum Medical Clinic in Santa Barbara has found that a nutrition bar called Balance controls blood sugar levels more effectively than the breakfast usually recommended for diabetics and hypoglycemics. Call 1-800-678-4246 for further information.

Hypothyroidism

One gland in particular that can start to act up around midlife is the thyroid gland, a member of the endocrine system of glands in the body. This small butterfly-shaped gland, located in the neck just below the Adams apple, works hand in hand with the adrenal glands to produce energy. Although it weighs less than 1 oz. and secretes less than 1 tsp. of thyroid hormone a year, it regulates the body's metabolism. The thyroid hormone, thyroxine, keeps all bodily processes operating, including heart rate, body temperature, muscle contraction, calorie use, protein synthesis, and production of the enzymes used to break down carbohydrates to glucose.

Thyroid problems are common, with some health professionals estimating that half of the U.S. adult population suffers from symptoms associated with low thyroid function, known as hypothyroidism. Women are five times more likely than men to suffer from low thyroid function, most commonly developing symptoms between the ages of 35 and 60. This may be because they are also more likely to have gone on extreme diet regimens, whereby the thyroid gland perceives the body to be going into a state of famine and cuts back on its production of thyroxine. Dr. Lawrence Wood, president and medical director of the Thyroid Foundation of America, states, "By the time a woman turns 50, she has about a one in eight chance of becoming hypothyroid."

It is also important to note that estrogen can decrease thyroid hormone uptake. It is not unusual for women on estrogen replacement to complain of tiredness and lack of energy—primary symptoms of hypothyroidism—when hormone tests are normal.

All bodily functions suffer from reduced energy metabolism when the thyroid stops producing enough thyroxine, or when the thyroxine is inactivated by yeast protein. Our bodily systems shift into low gear, resulting in a myriad of largely subtle and nonspecific symptoms. Although the most common complaint of people suffering from hypothyroidism is tiredness or chronic fatigue, symptoms may also include muscle weakness, stiffness, or cramping, loss of appetite accompanied by weight gain, joint aches and pains, headaches, nervousness, depression, memory loss, lowered body temperature, constipation, inability to concentrate, brittle hair and nails, and unusually light or heavy menstrual periods. A lack of thyroxine can also lead to elevated cholesterol and triglyceride levels, which in older women are high risk factors for heart disease. Individuals suffering from hypothyroidism are also prone to recurring infections anywhere in the body, because the lack of thyroxine leads to a sluggish immune system.

Stephen E. Langer, M.D., believes that nutritional imbalances contribute to the growing number of cases of hypothyroidism. Dr. Langer, who practices general preventive medicine and clinical nutrition in Berkeley, California, and is the author of *Solved: The Riddle of Illness,* also feels these nutritional imbalances have become more common as the American diet has become increasingly depleted of essential vitamins and minerals. In order to produce even the small amount of thyroid hormone used by the body each year, the thyroid must have a good supply of "raw material," and the typical American diet does not provide it.

Since menopause coincides with the onset of hypothyroidism in many women, symptoms of fatigue may be attributed to menopause while the underlying thyroid condition is ignored. This can further increase cancer risk, as thyroid function is related to unopposed estrogen production. Although we don't know why, it has been noted time and again that when thyroid hormone levels are low, estrogen levels tend to be high; high estrogen levels are known to increase a woman's risk for uterine and breast cancer. Low thyroid function may also be associated with problems in new bone formation, and in postmenopausal women, excessive use of synthetic thyroid medication can be a significant factor in bone loss. If you are taking thyroid medication, it would be wise to check with your doctor periodically to see if you can lower your dose or switch to a natural, desiccated thyroid. John R. Lee, M.D., suggests trying natural progesterone body cream which can enhance thyroid hormone activity. He states that women who are given natural progesterone often can reduce their dosage of thyroid medication.

An often overlooked factor in low thyroid function is systemic candidiasis. *Candida albicans* is a yeastlike fungus, naturally occurring in our bodies. *Candida* only becomes a problem when it grows out of control and out of balance with the bacteria in our bodies. Overgrowth of *Candida* is prevalent among women who have a history of antibiotic use, have been on estrogen-rich birth-control pills, have had children, and/or have been on high-sugar diets. It is estimated that one in three women harbor an overgrowth of *Candida.* According to Lendon H. Smith, M.D., in his book *Happiness Is a Healthy Life,* "The yeast protein of the candidiasis has receptor sites on it for both thyroid hormone and estrogen. That would help to explain why the laboratory would find the normal amount of thyroid hormone circulating about in the bloodstream; it is there and measurable but it is partially inactivated by its affinity to the yeast protein. The body is not receiving the benefits until the yeast is put under control."

Hypothyroidism, with its symptoms of fatigue, depression, nervousness, headaches, and inability to concentrate, is often misdiagnosed, in midlife women mistakenly attributed to menopause and/or "natural" signs of aging, and tranquilizers or antidepressants may be prescribed. Thyroid-induced elevated cholesterol and triglyceride levels may be misdiagnosed as primary heart disease and treated with estrogen-replacement therapy; recurring infections may be treated with repeated doses of antibiotics. Unfortunately, these treatments do not solve the problem, often making the underlying thyroid condition worse and adding new problems such as yeast overgrowth.

The standard blood tests used by most doctors to measure the two types of thyroxine in our bloodstream, T_3 and T_4, are not sensitive enough in many cases. One of the more accurate tests for thyroid function is the basal temperature test, developed by Broda O. Barnes, M.D., Ph.D., a pioneer in thyroid research, and author of *Hypothyroidism: The Unsuspected Illness*. This simple test involves taking the axillary (underarm) temperature for 10 minutes before rising, on two consecutive mornings. Because of temperature fluctuations during the menstrual cycle, women should take this test on the second and third days of their period. At night, before retiring, shake down a thermometer and lay it beside the bed on a night table or chair. On awakening in the morning— before getting out of bed—place the thermometer under your bare arm for 10 minutes. Record the temperature for 2 consecutive days. The temperature range for normal thyroid function is 97.8 to 98.2°F. A reading below this is strongly suggestive of low thyroid function. Readings above this may indicate infection or an overactive thyroid gland.

The Super Nutrition Approach for the Thyroid

Fortunately, nutrition can go a long way in helping the thyroid. Of all the raw materials used by the thyroid, you probably are familiar with iodine because it is the most well known, but there are many other nutrients, including the B vitamins (especially B_1), zinc, manganese, and the amino acids phenylalanine and tyrosine, that are essential for proper functioning of this important gland. The thyroid hormones manufactured in the body need both iodine and phenylalanine, which breaks down into tyrosine. Lack of either of these would cause a lack of thyroid hormones, resulting in the swelling of the thyroid gland, a condition known as a goiter. The common use of iodized salt has virtually eliminated goiters, but it has not eliminated the problem of low thyroid function. Low levels of zinc and phenylalanine have also been shown to reduce levels of thyroid hormones. I would suggest taking at least 25 mg of zinc on a daily basis for 1 month, then reducing to 15 mg for 3 times per week thereafter.

There are other minerals, such as calcium, magnesium, sodium, and potassium, that also help to regulate thyroid function. One of the best ways to find out which particular vitamins and minerals may be deficient is through a special test called a hair analysis, which measures tissue mineral levels. The hair, considered a storage organ, gives a better picture of underlying nutrient imbalances than the blood because it can reveal what has been going on in your body for several months.

Correcting underlying vitamin and mineral imbalances can do much to correct thyroid function without use of the synthetic hormones traditionally prescribed. We can all nourish the thyroid by eating vitamin B–rich foods such as wheat germ, whole grains, nuts, seeds, dark green leafy vegetables, and legumes. Brewer's yeast can be taken as a natural source of B vitamins. Kelp, dulse, and Irish moss seaweeds, as well as natural iodized salt, are good sources of sodium and iodine. Vitamin E is essential for increasing iodine absorption and can be taken along with it in the form of wheat germ oil (the richest natural source), unprocessed vegetable oils, or vitamin E supplements. I recommend 400 IU of vitamin E two to three times daily. Foods such as milk, meat, poultry, fish, legumes, nuts, eggs, bread, and cheese that are particularly concentrated in the amino acid phenylalanine will enhance hormone function. Natural progesterone cream can help enhance thyroid activity, too.

For those women taking synthetic thyroid hormones, certain foods containing thyroid-blocking substances should be limited. This also applies to women who suspect they have thyroid problems but are not on medication. These foods include soybeans, uncooked cabbage, cauliflower, mustard greens, turnips, Brussels sprouts, kale, and rutabaga. If *Candida* is present, limit all yeast-containing and fermented foods, alcohol, and sugar. Nourishing the thyroid, whether you are taking medication or not, will help to correct underlying vitamin and mineral imbalances and strengthen this primary gland. As you supplement nutritionally, your need for medication may decrease. Remember to check with your physician to make sure you are not overmedicating a condition that has been nutritionally corrected.

7
Prime-Time Exercise Prescription

Coupled with a balanced diet, exercise is the most important lifestyle habit for the midlife woman. In fact, Janine O'Leary Cobb, author of *Understanding Menopause,* and founder/publisher of the menopause newsletter, *A Friend Indeed,* states, "The best preparation for menopause is exercise—it helps keep weight down, handles stress, and reduces risk of osteoporosis and heart disease. If there's one thing a woman should do to prepare for menopause, it's exercise."

Exercise helps to strengthen bones, stimulates the formation of new bone, and aids in calcium metabolism. Activities that are aerobic provide intermittent stress and strain, which actually stretches the bone and helps to maintain and build bone mass. The stress causes an electric current to go through the bone, triggering the calcification process, known as the piezoelectric effect. An added bonus for the prime-time woman is that exercise can mobilize stored estrogen from the fatty tissue.

A word of caution: strenuous exercise should be avoided. For women in adrenal burn-out, exercising to exhaustion is counterproductive and puts more stress on the adrenals. Overexercise, like underexercise, can actually contribute to a calcium loss in a very thin woman. Too much exercise (over 2 hours of strenuous, nonstop activity on a daily basis) causes a halt in estrogen production—as in menopause—that can result in disrupted calcium metabolism. Even when exercise is decreased and estrogen levels become normalized, a 20 percent bone loss remains. If this cycle is repeated and the diet contains lots of calcium-robbers such as coffee, sugar, and soda, premature bone thinning will set in before menopause begins. It is important that balance be the key note in exercise, as in diet, during our twenties and thirties, before we reach our forties and fifties, when the bone-protecting benefits of estrogen begin to decline.

Overexercise can also lead to hormonal imbalance. Increased losses of body fat, brought on by strenuous exercise, first cause progesterone levels to drop. Progesterone deficiency may ensue, and this leads to bone loss. The secondary consequence of increased fat losses is the depletion of estrogen stores, resulting in menstrual irregularities, including cessation of menstrual periods. This situation is often evident in trained athletes such as body builders, runners, and ballet dancers, who can turn their periods on and off with a 3- to 5-lb. weight gain or loss. Women who were involved in athletics in their teens and twenties and missed at least one-third of their regular menstrual periods might be wise to check out their current bone density. In older women, this exercise-induced hormonal imbalance may be confused with menopause.

The answer is a balanced aerobic, weight-bearing exercise program that may include brisk walking, hiking, biking, rowing, tennis, other racquet sports, weightlifting, and jumping rope. Swimming would not be a good choice because it is not weight-bearing

—you're weightless in the water. Remember, weight-bearing exercise appears to be one vital element of the bone-building formula because bones become stronger with physical stress. If they're not used, they lose calcium and become porous.

Exercise is beneficial to the body in numerous ways. It brings blood, nutrients, and fresh oxygen to every cell in the body. It improves digestion, absorption, metabolism, and assimilation of food while increasing the efficiency of the body's enzyme reserves. For midlife women, it is a wonderful way of lowering blood fats while keeping the good HDL (high-density lipoprotein) cholesterol elevated. Tufts University researchers suggest that regular walking may even reverse osteoporosis. Most osteoporosis-prevention programs recommend a 30- to 40-minute brisk walk at least four times a week. For diabetics, exercise can lower blood sugar levels and make insulin more effective for your muscle and fat cells.

Regular exercise increases endurance, muscle tone and strength, flexibility, and disease resistance. The cardiovascular system is particularly benefited: as the lungs and heart become stronger, arteries become more resilient, blood pressure is lowered, and blood lipid levels of both cholesterol and triglycerides are controlled. Exercise is a strong weapon against strokes, atherosclerosis, phlebitis, and heart attacks because of increased oxygen flow. Joint problems such as bursitis and osteoarthritis can also be aided by stretching exercises.

The increased oxygen intake from aerobic exercise aids the brain and the complexion. It helps to alleviate nervous irritability, depression, and anxiety. It also relieves tiredness and increases energy. Resistance to the common cold is enhanced and sleep, weight loss, appetite control, and bowel regularity can be immeasurably improved. Cellular wastes are moved through the system for better elimination via the kidneys, bowels, and skin. Emotional health is also a by-product of regular exercise; a feeling of "centeredness" and well-being is often experienced by devotees of regular exercise. Exercise releases valuable endorphins, the brain's natural mood elevators, which contribute to feeling good and in control. Exercise may be the perfect prescription for those "menopause blues" that some women experience.

The Best Things in Life Are Free (or Almost)

The nice thing about most exercise is that it is available to everybody, practically any time of the year, at little or no cost. An ideal, well-rounded exercise program should include certain kinds of exercises designed to meet the three basic physical fitness components: cardiovascular endurance, muscle strength, and flexibility. Choosing a variety of exercises that fit into these categories will ensure that the entire body gets a workout. While some of the exercises can be done at gyms and studios, they can also be done at home alone or with family and friends or your television set!

The cardiovascular activities known as aerobic exercises include swimming, bike riding, rowing, cross-country skiing, brisk walking, jogging, racquet sports, jumping rope, and aerobic dancing. What all of these activities have in common is that they require a sustained supply of oxygen for long periods of time.

This conditions the heart and respiratory system, pumping oxygen to all parts of the body. For these exercises to be effective, you must sustain them, keeping up your pulse rate for 15 to 30 minutes. Cardiovascular exercises promote energy and endurance, and raise the level of the "happy hormones" in the bloodstream.

For muscle endurance, the best choices include weight training, progressive resistance training on Nautilus machinery, pushups and situps. These exercises help tighten and tone the muscles, aiding weight loss because building muscle tissue uses more calories than fat tissue. In addition to building muscle, these exercises build stronger bones, and strong, healthy bones are the best prevention for osteoporosis.

Flexibility exercises can be chosen from yoga, ballet, modern dance, and special stretch and tone classes offered at many fitness and dance studios. Good for combating muscle and joint stiffness, these exercises make us bend, extend, and stretch. Besides alleviating physical tightness, flexibility exercises can help release stress and tension.

While working on this book, I found myself in great need of an easy flexibility exercise program. Because I was so engrossed with my work, I was sitting for long periods of time and found myself becoming stiff and tight, particularly in my lower back. I started special classes for the Pilates method, a conditioning program designed to improve muscle control, coordination, strength, and tone. The exercise program (on mats and machines) not only helped relieve my lower back pain, but has helped my posture and strengthened my abdominal and back muscles. I now use a Pilates video every morning for stretching and warm-up.

The Pilates method is particularly effective for menopausal women. It builds bone mass without the stress of gravity, and Kegel principles (as discussed in Chapter 1) are utilized so that incontinence, prolapsed uterus, and bulging abdominals are avoided. Long, lean muscles are developed, so Pilates devotees look slimmer. Finally, because breathing patterns are coupled with the variety of movements, a Pilates work-out leaves you destressed, relaxed, and balanced.

For women who have not been exercising on a regular basis, here is a sample weekly program that you can follow:

- Cardiovascular exercises: 3 days a week (for at least 30 minutes each day)
- Muscle strength exercises: in alternation with cardiovascular exercises, 3 days a week (for at least 30 minutes each day)
- Flexibility exercises: daily (for at least 20 minutes)

My own schedule includes aerobic dancing three times a week for cardiovascular endurance, free weights three times a week, and my Pilates video every morning for flexibility. For information on the Pilates method, write to the Pilates Institute, Ltd., 1802 Second Street, #28, Santa Fe, NM 87501, or call 1-505-988-1990.

'Tis the Season

There are combinations of cardiovascular, muscle strength, and flexibility exercises that can be enjoyed seasonally. When the weather permits, it is distinctly more beneficial to exercise outside because of the added health bonus of sunlight. As previously discussed, the sun's rays aid in vitamin D production, which is critical to calcium absorption. It also provides stimulation to the optic nerve, which tonifies every gland in the body. Full-spectrum light from the sun also alleviates the cyclical mood-change syndrome known as Seasonal Affective Disorder (SAD), a kind of depression that is characterized by lethargy and overeating. The light–hormone connection is well worth investigating if you have been suffering these problems, particularly in winter. If sunlight is not easily available, then you might want to purchase full-spectrum lights for application indoors. These lights are sold by the Duro-Test Corporation in North Bergen, New Jersey.

The following chart lists the most suitable exercises for the different seasons and climates. If you have year-round access to health clubs, then include swimming and exercises for muscle strength as part of your total exercise plan.

Spring: running, jogging, tennis, volleyball, badminton, stretching exercises or dance classes, roller skating

Summer: walking/hiking, swimming, rowing, water skiing

Autumn: brisk aerobic walking, bicycling, jumping rope, martial arts, stretching and toning exercises

Winter: cross-country skiing, yoga, ice skating, tai chi, breath control

Wet Climate: indoor sports, low-impact aerobics, stretching and toning exercises, walking

Dry Climate: Walking, low impact aerobics, stretch and tone exercises.

Gain Without Pain: Warm-Ups and Cool-Downs

A series of warm-up exercises for 5 to 10 minutes is a good way to slowly ease into your exercise program. The purpose of these warm-ups is to limber muscles, to increase blood flow to all body parts, and to deepen your breathing for full exercise benefits. Light stretching, yoga postures, or calisthenics can prevent stiff muscles later on. Warming up the muscles is important so as to avoid injury and to prevent muscle soreness, which could prevent you from continuing your exercise program. The same warm-up series of movements can be applied to cool-downs for 5 to 10 minutes after the vigorous part of your exercise is completed. If you do not have time for both, the warm-ups are the most important.

Seasonal Shifts

In the warm weather of spring or summer or in dry climates, drink water before exercising to replace fluids that will be lost in perspiration. The rule of thumb is a quart of water to 100 lbs. of body weight. Some fitness buffs feel best when they drink a glass of water on the hour to ensure sufficient hydration of body tissue. Some of the bottled mineral waters, such as Evian, are high in magnesium and potassium, which helps to balance body fluids.

In cold weather you must also drink a lot of water because urine output triples in volume when the weather is cold. As in hot temperature conditions, water can hydrate body tissue and will also help keep a steady body temperature. Remember to do your warm-up exercises indoors before exercising outdoors; this will acclimate your body to stressful cold temperatures.

For hot-weather fitness and health, cotton clothing is your best bet. Lightweight materials that can easily absorb perspiration and then dry quickly are advisable. Try to avoid antiperspirants, which block sweating, the body's natural cooling mechanism. This is particularly important for menopausal women who are experiencing hot flashes or night sweats.

In cold weather, clothing should be loose rather than tight-fitting. Choose the layered look, consisting of several layers of natural material. Insulation is provided through the warm air-filled spaces between the layers. Plastic fabrics or polyester should be avoided because these fabrics do not allow the skin to breathe, a special concern for the prime-time woman. Do remember to keep your head and neck covered to protect body heat from escaping. Also, try to stay dry. Melting snow and rain create moisture, affecting clothing insulation. Water removes body heat at least 20 times faster than air.

Consistency Is the Key

The ultimate key to exercise is regularity. Many individuals make exercise a part of their daily regimen. Others exercise 4 days out of 7 to keep the blood moving, muscles toned, and joints flexible. Whatever you decide to do, approach your program realistically and with joy. Exercise is a lifelong activity, so avoid crash programs, which can be painful and dangerous in the long run.

The Lymphatic System: Rebounding for Health

My own personal exercise regimen also includes daily use of the mini-trampoline. This little rebounder helps to exercise the lymphatics, a secondary circulation system we don't seem to hear as much about in the United States. The lymphatic system rids the body of toxic wastes, bacteria, heavy metals, dead cells, trapped protein, and fatty globules. In essence, the lymphatic system is the garbage disposal of the body. All waste material and immune cells—called lymphocytes—are circulated and stored in the lymphatic system before removal through the elimination organs. The lymphatic system pumps only through muscular action via the thighs and arms. The heart does not move the lymph as it does the bloodstream. It is important to exercise the lymphatic drainage system for total cellular cleansing. No matter where you live, you can exercise the lymphatics by bouncing on a mini-trampoline and rebounder for 5 to 20 minutes a day.

The mini-trampoline has proved to be one of the most efficient, yet least harmful, forms of exercise. A high level of cardiovascular fitness and toning results from regular bouncing every day. The low-impact rebounding acts to gently move the waste materials in the lymph. Most people must start slowly and bounce for only 5 minutes at a time, then work up slowly until they are jumping for the suggested 20-minute span. The light pressure on the thighs of jumping activates lymphatic drainage. Within 2 weeks, legs, buttocks, and ankles are toned and fatty cellulite deposits begin to disappear.

The advantage of the mini-trampoline is its universality. It can be used by people of all ages, in all stages of life. Even handicapped people who cannot walk can sit on it or put their feet on it while someone else is bouncing and still receive lymphatic benefits.

For a more strenuous work-out, simply jump faster and lower. Bouncing is the exercise par excellence for all seasons and climates. The mini-trampoline is portable, versatile, and requires no instruction. Every home should have one!

8
The Prime-Time Diet

The Prime-Time Supernutrition Plan features the right fats, high levels of complex carbohydrates, mineral-rich fruits and vegetables, and quality protein, all in moderation and balance. This diet is specifically designed for a woman's unique needs at menopause, as a key in protecting against heart disease, cancer, osteoporosis, and can make you feel and look better overall. After working with so many women for so many years, I realize that a drastic change in eating habits can be overwhelming. Because we are faced with so many new body conditions at menopause to begin with, this is not the time to make dietary changes all at once. You can make changes step by step and find better food choices for what you will be limiting or eliminating, such as replacing coffee with herbal teas. I know you can do it because I've seen all of my clients make improvements in diet without changing eating habits drastically.

General Prime-Time Dietary Guidelines

Beverages

I have found that changing what you drink is a good first step toward better health. Avoid coffee, regular tea, soda pop, and excessive amounts of alcohol because of their effects on calcium, magnesium, and the stress-fighting B vitamins. Coffee and alcohol also exert a dehydrating effect on body tissue. Remember—alcohol is implicated in every negative health condition covered in this book (heart disease, low adrenals, diabetes, osteoporosis, and all the uncomfortable symptoms of menopause), however, limited amounts—2 to 4 ounces—may actually improve HDL/cholesterol ratios and lower incidence of cardiovascular disease.

The best beverage of all is clear, pure, noncarbonated water. Water helps rid the body of waste, keeps tissues moist and lubricated, and can help burn calories. A mere 5 percent loss of body moisture causes skin shrinkage and muscle weakness, just what we *don't* need at this time of life. I suggest drinking purified or bottled water from a reliable source or a water filter for your home.

Herbal teas, drunk hot or cold, are good substitutes for sodas and coffee. In addition to containing no caffeine, many of these pleasant-tasting teas (such as rose hips, chamomile, and hibiscus) contain surprising amounts of vitamins and minerals. Try grain-based coffee substitutes such as Pero, Roma, Caffix, and Sipp.

Prime-Time Oils

You will note that the Prime-Time Diet is a whole-some plan that includes, rather than excludes, vital amounts of naturally unprocessed oils as an essential part of the program. As previously discussed, oils provide essential fatty acids (EFAs), which are of prime importance at menopause because they nourish dry skin, hair, and mucous membranes as well as aid in natural hormone production. Oil also helps in the transport of calcium into the soft tissues. The four Prime-Time oils—flax seed, sesame, olive, and canola—can be used year-round in no-heat recipes and cooking. These oils are included for their delicious nutty flavors, beneficial fatty acids, and stability at high temperatures.

Unnatural fats, such as margarine, vegetable short-ening, and processed and hydrogenated vegetable oils, should be avoided. Omit highly saturated sources of fat such as palm and coconut oils (you'll need to read labels, as these oils are still abundant in prepared foods).

Protein

Rely more on poultry, fish, beans, legumes, and soy proteins (tofu and tempeh). Moderate amounts (3½ oz.) of lean red meat from beef and lamb can be included up to twice a week. These are good sources of readily available iron, zinc, and vitamin B_{12}, nutrients commonly deficient in a woman's diet. Eggs are also a good source of minerals. They can be used in modera-tion, up to four a week. Try to increase vegetable protein sources such as beans, nuts, and seeds.

To avoid secondhand hormones, buy naturally

raised beef, chicken, and turkey. Shelton Farms, Harmony Farms, Foster Farms, and Young Farm offer organically raised poultry, and Coleman Natural Beef is a source for organic beef. Look for these in your supermarket or your natural-food store. If currently unavailable in your area, ask your supermarket to order these organic meats for you.

Dairy Products

Due to the magnesium–calcium interaction, limit intake of high-calcium dairy products. I recommend two portions per day, maximum. The Lifetime natural part-skim cheeses are reduced at least 50 percent in fat, calories, and salt. No matter which dairy products you select, one portion equals 1 cup nonfat milk, 1 cup nonfat yogurt, or a half cup non- or low-fat cottage cheese.

Fruits and Vegetables

In keeping with the National Cancer Institute's "Five A Day" campaign, try to have at least five servings of fruits and vegetables per day. A vegetable serving is usually a half cup cooked or 1 cup raw. Each serving contains 2 to 3 g of fiber. I recommend fresh vegetables and fruits. Try to buy certified organic produce whenever possible. When unavailable, use frozen. Canned fruits and vegetables are least desirable, due to the salt added in the processing.

Brightly colored orange and yellow vegetables, such as carrots, yams, squash, and sweet potatoes, are high in the cancer-protecting beta carotene. Green foods are magnesium and vitamin A–rich. Bok choy, broccoli, kale, and sea vegetables are delicious sources of nondairy calcium. Remember, sea vegetables are also high in hard-to-find iron and trace minerals.

With the big interest in juicing these days, it is important to monitor intake. A glass of carrot juice generally contains four to five carrots without the dietary fiber, which slows down absorption of sugar. Carrots have a very high glycemic index, which means that in the form of juice, they can increase blood sugar levels very quickly. I recommend not drinking more than a quarter cup or 2 fluid oz. at one time.

Many women eat too many fruits in the mistaken belief that because they are natural they can be eaten without limits. Too much fruit, no matter what the source, can upset the delicate calcium balance in the system and increase triglyceride levels. If yeast problems are a concern, temporarily avoid all fruits for at least 10 days or eat just one fruit a day. Serving portions for fruit can be found in Table 8-1 (pages 146–47).

Complex Carbohydrates

Three or more servings per day from this family of foods is recommended. Serving portions for complex carbohydrates can be found in Table 8-2 (pages 148–51). Fiber-rich grains like buckwheat, millet, and barley are particularly recommended for their high magnesium content. Whole unprocessed grains and legumes are good nonanimal protein and iron sources. Dried beans, peas, and lentils are tops in high fiber, with from 4 to 8 g per serving.

For women who are wheat or gluten sensitive, there are two grains on the menus that are great alternatives —amaranth and quinoa. These grains have a buttery

Table 8-1
Serving Portions for Fruit

Fruit	Serving Portion
Apple	1 small (2-in. diameter)
Apple butter (sugar-free)	2 tbsp.
Apple juice or cider	$\frac{1}{3}$ cup
Applesauce (unsweetened)	$\frac{1}{2}$ cup
Apricots (fresh)	2 medium
Apricots (dried and unsulphured)	4 halves
Banana	One-half small
Berries: boysenberries, blackberries, blueberries, loganberries, raspberries	$\frac{1}{2}$ cup
Cantaloupe	One-quarter (6-in. diameter)
Cherries	10 large
Dates	2
Figs (fresh)	1 large
Figs (dried)	1 small
Fruit cocktail (canned in juice)	$\frac{1}{2}$ cup
Fruit preserves and spreads (sugar-free)	2 tbsp.
Grapefruit	One-half small
Grapefruit juice	$\frac{1}{2}$ cup
Grapes	12
Grape juice	$\frac{1}{4}$ cup

Fruit	Serving Portion
Honeydew melon	One-eighth (7-in. diameter)
Mandarin oranges (canned)	$\frac{3}{4}$ cup
Kiwi	1 medium
Mango	One-half small
Nectarine	1 small
Orange	1 small
Orange juice (any style)	$\frac{1}{2}$ cup
Papaya	$\frac{3}{4}$ cup
Peach	1 medium
Pear	1 small
Persimmon	1 medium
Pineapple	$\frac{1}{2}$ cup
Pineapple juice	$\frac{1}{3}$ cup
Plums	2 medium
Prunes	2 medium
Prune juice	$\frac{1}{4}$ cup
Raisins	2 tbsp.
Strawberries	$\frac{3}{4}$ cup
Tangerine	1 large
Watermelon	1 cup

(Adapted from Gittleman, AL: *Supernutrition for Women,* Bantam, New York, 1991, with permission.)

Table 8-2
Serving Portions for Carbohydrates

Food	Serving Portion
Starchy Vegetables	
Chestnuts, roasted	4 large or 6 small
Corn (on the cob)	1 (4 in. long)
Corn (cooked)	$\frac{1}{3}$ cup
Parsnips	1 small
Peas (fresh)	$\frac{1}{4}$ cup
Potatoes, white (baked or boiled)	1 small
Potatoes, white (mashed)	$\frac{1}{2}$ cup
Pumpkin	$\frac{3}{4}$ cup
Rutabaga	1 small
Squash (winter types)	$\frac{1}{2}$ cup
Succotash	$\frac{1}{2}$ cup
Breads	
Bagel, whole wheat	$\frac{1}{2}$ small
Bread (rye, pumpernickel, whole wheat)	1 slice
Breadsticks	4 (7 in. long)
Bun (hamburger or hot dog)	One-half
Croutons	$\frac{1}{2}$ cup
English muffin	One-half
Pancakes	2 (3-in. diameter)

Food	Serving Portion
Pita bread	One-half (6-inch pocket)
Rice cakes	2
Roll	1 (2-in. diameter)

Cereals and Grains

Food	Serving Portion
Amaranth (cooked)	$\frac{1}{2}$ cup
Barley (cooked)	$\frac{1}{2}$ cup
Bran flakes	$\frac{1}{2}$ cup
Bran (unprocessed rice or wheat)	$\frac{1}{2}$ cup
Buckwheat groats (kasha, cooked)	$\frac{1}{2}$ cup
Cornmeal (cooked)	$\frac{1}{2}$ cup
Couscous	$\frac{1}{2}$ cup
Cream of rice (cooked)	$\frac{1}{2}$ cup
Grapenuts	$\frac{1}{4}$ cup
Grits (cooked)	$\frac{1}{2}$ cup
Kamut	$\frac{1}{2}$ cup
Millet (cooked)	$\frac{1}{2}$ cup
Oatmeal	$\frac{1}{2}$ cup
Popcorn	3 cups
Puffed rice, wheat, millet, or oats	$1\frac{1}{2}$ cups
Quinoa (cooked)	$\frac{1}{2}$ cup
Rice (brown, cooked)	$\frac{1}{3}$ cup
Rice (wild, cooked)	$\frac{1}{2}$ cup

Table 8-2 *(con't)*

Food	Serving Portion
Shredded-wheat biscuit	1 large
Spelt	$\frac{1}{2}$ cup
Tapioca	2 tbsp.
Wheatena (cooked)	$\frac{1}{2}$ cup
Wheat germ	1 oz. or 3 tbsp.

Crackers

Matzoh (whole wheat)	$\frac{1}{2}$ (6 × 4 in.)
Pretzels (whole grain)	1 large
Rice wafers (brown rice, Westbrae)	4
Rye crispbread cracker (Wasa)	$1\frac{1}{2}$ crackers
Whole wheat crackers (AK-Mak)	4 crackers
Whole Wheat Crackers (Health Valley)	13 crackers

Flours

Arrowroot	2 tbsp.
Buckwheat	3 tbsp.
Cornmeal	3 tbsp.
Cornstarch	2 tbsp.
Potato flour	$2\frac{1}{2}$ tbsp.
Rice flour	3 tbsp.
Soya powder	3 tbsp.
Whole wheat	3 tbsp.

Food	Serving Portion
Legumes	
Beans: lima, navy, pinto, kidney, garbanzos, black (dried, cooked)	$\frac{1}{2}$ cup
Beans (baked, plain)	$\frac{1}{2}$ cup
Lentils (dried, cooked)	$\frac{1}{2}$ cup
Peas (dried, cooked)	$\frac{1}{2}$ cup
Pasta	
Noodles: macaroni, spaghetti (cooked)	$\frac{1}{2}$ cup
Noodles: rice (cooked)	$\frac{1}{2}$ cup
Noodles: (whole wheat, cooked)	$\frac{1}{2}$ cup
Pasta: (whole wheat, cooked)	$\frac{1}{2}$ cup

(Adapted from Gittleman, AL: *Supernutrition for Women*, Bantam, New York, 1991, with permission.)

rich flavor. Amaranth, a tiny grain seed that is a fairly new addition to store shelves, was widely used by the Aztecs in Mexico hundreds of years ago and was revered as a magical, mystical grain. It is one of the highest protein grains at 20 percent. A half-cup serving also has as much calcium as an 8-oz. glass of milk. Amaranth is a good source of lysine and methionine, essential amino acids lacking in almost all other grains. This unusual grain can be used alone as a cereal or added to the batter of breads and baked goods. Quinoa is reputed to be as high or higher in protein value than amaranth. Known as the "mother grain" of the Incas, quinoa is low in gluten but is an abundant source of the amino acids methionine and cystine as well as lysine. Both of these grains are used as cereals and flour and are available without pesticides or sprays. Avoid all white-flour products.

Seasonings

High sodium intake may be connected to high blood pressure, stroke, and heart and kidney disease. The first thing to do is cut all processed foods, such as chips, dips, and fast foods, out of the diet. Practically two-thirds of the sodium in the diet comes from these sources. Try to keep sodium intake to no more than 2,000 to 3,000 mg per day. I recommend using Real Salt, an unrefined sea salt that does not have any additives. (Commercial salt is chemically cleaned, has added aluminum silicate to prevent caking and dextrose to cover up the bitterness of the aluminum.) Try substituting garlic or onion powder, kelp, dill, parsley, thyme, and cayenne. Remember that the very hot spices, such as curries and chili peppers, encourage water retention.

Healthy Fast Food

Sometimes no matter how hard we try, we just can't find time to eat. Balance is a healthy nutrition bar that provides high-quality protein, carbohydrates, and good fat. To order Balance bars, call 1-800-678-4246.

Cooking Utensils

It is best to avoid *all* aluminum-containing pots, pans, and foil because aluminum hampers the body's utilization of calcium and phosphorus. High-quality stainless steel, cast iron, enamel-covered iron, Corning Wear, Pyrex, and glass are preferable. I use Royal Prestige cookware, which features the minimum–moisture method so that food cooks without a lot of extra water or fats. For more information on this system, call 1-800-888-4353

The real danger of aluminum comes from the aluminum hydroxides in many antacids, in baking powder and baking soda and the fluoride that is in aluminum foil. If you are going to freeze or refigerate in aluminum foil, it is best to first wrap with waxed paper, and then use the aluminum, so that none will leach into your food.

Nutritional Supplementation

As a nutritionist, I believe—and I know my clients believe—that food is our best source of vitamins, minerals, enzymes, and amino acids for health. But due to hectic schedules, we can't always eat the way we know we should. Plus, topsoil is now depleted in certain trace minerals, such as zinc, chromium, selenium, and magnesium, that are important more now than ever for health. The stress of modern-day life, environmental pollution, and radiation all take their nutrient tolls on the twentieth-century body. Supplemental vitamins and minerals have become a necessity, not a luxury. It is no wonder that over 80 million Americans are now supplementing their diets.

In light of these situational constraints and the major glandular shifts occurring at midlife, Rejuvex, a one-day caplet available at most drugstores, is recommended. For my clients I recommend a special comprehensive regimen to help fulfill their unique nutritional needs:

- Natural Progesterone Body Cream: ¼ to ½ tsp. 2 times a day
- Osteo Forte: 1 tablet 3 times a day
- Magnesium Forte: 1 tablet once a day (separate from Osteo Forte)
- Vitamin E: 400 IU 3 times a day (for a total of 1,200 IU)
- Vitamin B complex: 50 mg 3 times a day (for a total of 150 mg)
- Super Nutrition Energy Formula (adrenal and stress support): 2 tablets 3 times a day (for a total of 6 tablets)
- Digestive Compound (hydrochloric acid and pepsin for digestive support): 2 tablets 3 times a day (for a total of 6 tablets)
- Avail's Vitase Plant Enzyme: 2–4 capsules 3 times a day before meals
- Super Oils (essential fatty acids source): 2 capsules 2 times a day (for a total of 4 tablets)
- Avail's Meno-Fem (gamma-oryzanol source): 1–2 capsules 2 times a day

For my diabetic clients and those who crave sugar I add 200 mcg of chromium, two times per day.

These supplements can be ordered directly from Uni Key at 1-800-888-4353. Do remember that individual requirements may vary.

Mindful Medicine

Prescription drugs and over-the-counter medications can interfere with the digestion and absorption of key nutrients. Antibiotics and antacids affect calcium utilization. Diuretics eliminate potassium, zinc, and magnesium. Potassium is often prescribed with water pills, but zinc and magnesium are not—two minerals in short supply to begin with.

Aspirin interferes with vitamin C and iron absorption, and can also magnify the effects of other medications, such as blood thinners. If you are taking prescription drugs, try to eat foods high in the vitamins that the medication depletes or consider vitamin supplementation. Table 8-3 (pages 161-64) gives a listing of commonly prescribed drugs and their interactions with key nutrients.

Even foods interact with drugs. Milk interferes with the absorption of certain antibiotics, such as tetracycline. Aged cheese, bananas, soy sauce, sour cream, and Chianti wine should not be taken with a monoamine oxydase (MAO) inhibitor, used to control high blood pressure. This combination can increase blood pressure to dangerously high levels, which could result in brain hemorrhage and death. Carbohydrates such as bread and crackers increase the time it takes for some over-the-counter pain relievers, like Tylenol, to take affect.

It is helpful to know about drug interactions, so as to avoid reactions. Make sure that your primary physician is aware of every single prescription drug and over-the-counter medication you are taking. (In this age of medical specialists, it is common for people to see different physicians for different health concerns, getting medications from each doctor, none of whom may be aware of the other's prescriptions.) Some drugs can cancel out the effect of others, magnify potency, or reduce their effects. You should know all potential side effects, whether your medicine should be taken with meals or without food, and the length of time you should be on it.

Putting It All Together

Here's an easy-to-follow list of the Prime-Time Diet daily recommendations:

Beverages: 8 glasses of pure, fresh water, taken plain or used to make herbal beverages

Oils: 2 tbsp. of Prime-Time Oils

Protein: 6 oz. (preferably poultry, fish, soy or legumes)

Dairy products: 2 nonfat servings

Fruits and vegetables: 5 or more servings

Complex carbohydrates: 3 or more servings

Throughout this book I have made a lot of food suggestions. The menus at the end of this chapter put them all together, based on a seasonal overview because most of our eating patterns are dictated by what's available seasonally. Fresh raw fruits and vegetables are more prevalent in our summer menus when they are readily available not only at the supermarket but in our gardens. More warming foods, such as soups, beans, cooked grains, and root vegetables, tend to predominate our winter fare. As Perla Meyer, author of *The Seasonal Kitchen,* says, "Seasonal cooking is catching freshness at its prime."

The menu plans introduce several exotic-sounding foods that have special health benefits for women. You may not choose to use these foods, but they have been included because they are particularly high in minerals such as calcium, magnesium, and the essential fatty acids (EFAs), and contain healing properties for the female body. The root vegetables daikon and burdock that are featured in the autumn and winter menus are frequently used in oriental cooking. Daikon is a long white radish that assists digestion and metabolization of fats. Burdock, a medicinal root vegetable, is well respected for its blood-building and purifying properties.

Sesame seed paste, known as tahini, is included as a year-round shopping-list item because of its delightful taste and very high calcium content. Miso is a fermented soybean product that is a versatile cooking ingredient and is becoming quite popular in vegetarian cooking. It is especially noteworthy because it strengthens the blood and lymph and is a good source of enzymes, calcium, and iron. Tamari, an aged soy sauce, is another year-round item that is used in limited amounts as a flavorful alternative to salt and aids in digestion. Tofu and tempeh are soy products that are nonanimal sources of good-quality protein. Kuzu is a thickening agent similar to arrowroot but is higher in minerals, particularly iron.

You will see many varieties of sea vegetables in the recipes. These vegetables have absorbed nutrients from the sea and are chock-full of hard-to-find trace minerals, as well as the more common calcium and iron (it has 10 times more iron than spinach). Their nutritional qualities reach far beyond their rich mineral and vitamin content; most sea vegetables contain an element called sodium alginate that inhibits the absorption of radioactive and heavy-metal toxins. Sea vegetables are very versatile and can be used to flavor stews, spike soups, and enhance grains. The following list describes each vegetable and gives some suggestions for its preparation:

Hijiki tastes a bit like licorice and looks like tangled black strings. A half cup of cooked hijiki has almost the same calcium content as a half cup of milk. This vegetable should be rinsed in cold water and then soaked for 20 minutes. It can be added to soups or salads and is delicious sautéed with carrots and fresh ginger.

Wakame is a delicately flavored dark green leaf. It is a rich source of vitamins A, B complex, and E. It should be rinsed in cold water and soaked for 15 minutes. Add it to soups or dressings, or serve atop fish.

Kombu is a kelp with a sweet/salty flavor that is an excellent source of minerals such as magnesium, calcium, potassium, iron, and iodine. It can be toasted in the oven for snacks, added to beans to aid in digestion, or crumbled and sprinkled over fish, chicken, or rice dishes. Cut into strips, it can be added to soups.

Nori (green laver or sea lettuce) is a nutty-tasting seaweed, high in the B vitamins and vitamin A. Nori comes in sheets that can be toasted and crumbled over vegetables, pasta, or fish. The sheets can also be used untoasted to wrap other foods.

Arame is one of the milder tasting sea vegetables and would be a good one to use when introducing your tastebuds to sea vegetables. Arame is high in iron, calcium, potassium, and vitamins A and B. It should be rinsed in cool water and soaked for 10 to 15 minutes. (Soaking will cause it to more than double in size.) It makes a tasty addition to salads, soups, brown rice, and vegetables. Both hijiki and arame can be sautéed for 2 to 3 minutes in oil.

Agar agar is a seaweed that is sold in flake form to be used in place of gelatin for thickening puddings, molds, and mousses. Agar Agar is a high fiber vegetable that is soothing to the digestive tract.

Sea palm fronds are another mineral-rich treasure. This variety of sea vegetation is my particular favorite because when cooked, sea palm resembles green pasta ribbons. The taste is mild and it lends itself well to enhancing many dishes.

Beginning on page 165 are suggested seasonal shopping lists for adding diversity through knowledge of what is available fresh each season. You may want to refer to the list of Prime-Time Diet daily recommendations (on page 156) and then go to the shopping lists to select items and plan menus. I have also included one-week sample menu plans and recipes for each season based on a woman's unique nutritional needs. You will note that most of the recipes serve six. I did this so you could use these recipes at get-togethers and so there would be leftovers for freezing. The recipes may sound a bit exotic at first, but once you get used to the new flavors and foods, you may find you actually prefer them to your old diet.

Table 8-3
Drug and Nutrient Interactions

Drug Trade Name	Major Indication(s) for Use	Effect on Nutrient(s)
Achromycin	Gram-negative and gram-positive microorganisms	Reduces absorption of calcium, magnesium, and iron
Aldactazide	Hypertension, congestive heart failure, edema, diuretic action needed	Reduces potassium excretion
Aldactone	Hypertension, congestive heart failure, edema, diuretic action needed	Reduces potassium excretion
Apresoline	Hypertension	Depletes vitamin B_6
Aspirin	Minor pain	Causes deficiency in thiamin and vitamin C
Atromid-S	Cholesterol control	Reduces circulating vitamin K levels
Azo Gantanol	Antibacterial, gram-negative and gram-positive urinary tract infection	Causes deficiency in folic acid
Bentyl with phenobarbital	Functional gastrointestinal disorders, dizziness	Accelerates vitamin K metabolism
Brevicon	Oral contraception	Vitamin B_6 and C depletion
Bronkotabs and Bronkolixir	Bronchial asthma, bronchitis, emphysema	Accelerates vitamin K metabolism
Butazolidin	Rheumatoid arthritis and osteoarthritis, spondylitis	Causes deficiency in folic acid
Cantil with phenobarbital	Lower gastrointestinal distress, diarrhea, abdominal pain, cramping, irritable colon	Accelerates vitamin K metabolism

Table 8-3 *(con't)*

Drug Trade Name	Major Indication(s) for Use	Effect on Nutrient(s)
Chardonna	Nervous indigestion, gastritis, nausea, vomiting, spastic colon, flatulence	Accelerates vitamin K metabolism
Colchicine	Chronic gouty arthritis	Decreased absorption of lactase, fat, sodium, potassium, and B_{12}
Cortisone Tablets and Suspension	Adrenocortical deficiency, allergic states, rheumatoid arthritis, dermatoses	Causes deficiency in vitamin B_6, zinc, potassium, and vitamin C; accelerates vitamin D metabolism
Cortisporin	Acid deficiency, burns, wounds, skin grafts, otitis externa, eczema	Reduces levels of lactase, vitamins K and B_{12}, and folic acid
Diethylstilbestrol	Menopause, senile vaginitis	Depletes vitamin B_6
Demulen	Oral contraception	Depletes vitamins B_6 and C
Diupres	Hypertension	Increases magnesium and potassium excretion
Diuril	Hypertension	Increases potassium and magnesium excretion
Doriden	Insomnia	Causes deficiency in folic acid
Enovid	Oral contraception	Depletes vitamins B_6 and C
Gantanol	Urinary tract, soft tissue, and respiratory infections	Causes deficiency in folic acid
Indocin	Rheumatoid arthritis, spondylitis, degenerative joint or hip disease, gout	Depletes thiamin and vitamin C

Drug Trade Name	Major Indication(s) for Use	Effect on Nutrient(s)
Isordil with phenobarbital	Angina pectoris	Accelerates vitamin K metabolism
Lo-Oval	Oral contraception	Depletes vitamin B_6
Mycifradin	Enterocolitis and diarrhea	Reduces lactase levels, causes vitamin K deficiency and malabsorption of vitamin B_{12} and folic acid
Mycolog	Cutaneous candidiasis, infantile eczema	Reduces lactase levels, causes vitamin K deficiency and malabsorption of vitamin B_{12} and folic acid
Neo-Cortef	Contact and allergic dermatitis	Reduces lactase levels, causes vitamin K deficiency and malabsorption of vitamin B_{12} and folic acid
Neomycin	Suppression of intestinal bacteria, diarrhea	Reduces lactase levels, causes vitamin K deficiency and malabsorption of vitamin B_{12} and folic acid
Neosporin	*Pseudomonas, Staphylococcus* bacteria	Reduces lactase levels, causes vitamin K deficiency and malabsorption of vitamin B_{12} and folic acid
Norinyl	Oral contraception, hypermenorrhea, rheumatoid arthritis	Depletes vitamins B_6 and C, increases vitamin B_6 requirement

Table 8-3 (con't)

Drug Trade Name	Major Indication(s) for Use	Effect on Nutrient(s)
Os-Cal	Osteoporosis	Depletes vitamin B6
Phazyme	Gastrointestinal disturbances, aerophagia, dyspepsia, diverticulitis, spastic colitis	Accelerates vitamin K metabolism
Polysporin	Gram-negative and gram-positive microorganisms	Causes malabsorption of vitamins B12, K, and folic acid
Prednisone	Rheumatoid arthritis; joint pain, stiffness, swelling, and tenderness; asthma	Increases vitamin B6 requirement, increased vitamin C excretion, causes zinc, potassium, and calcium deficiency
Premarin	Menopausal syndrome, senile vaginitis, pruritis vulvae	Causes folic acid deficiency, reduces calcium excretion
Pro-Banthine	Peptic ulcer, hypertrophic gastritis, pancreatitis, diverticulitis	Accelerates vitamin K metabolism
Ser Ap-Es	Hypertension	Depletes vitamin B6
Sumycin	Gram-negative and gram-positive microorganisms	Reduces absorption of calcium, magnesium, and iron
Tetracyn	Gram-negative and gram-positive microorganisms	Reduces absorption of calcium, magnesium, and iron

Spring Diet

(Mid-March to Mid-June)

Herbs and Spices of Spring
Oregano, dill, basil, tarragon, marjoram, mint, parsley, chives, thyme, sorrel, chervil

Herb Teas for Spring
Chamomile, peppermint, linden, comfrey leaf

Shopping List

Spring Produce
Apples (Golden Delicious, Red Delicious, MacIntosh, Newtown Pippin, Rome Beauty, Granny Smith)

Artichokes

Asparagus

Beans (green, wax, Italian)

Broccoli

Brussels sprouts

Cabbage (red, green, Chinese or bok choy)

Carrots

Celery

Cucumbers

Garlic

Lemons

Mushrooms (wild: chanterelle, morel)

Onions (green, scallions, leeks, shallots, chives)

Oranges

Radishes

Rhubarb

Salad greens (Belgian endive, escarole, spinach, arugula, radicchio, watercress, parsley, and lettuces such as butter-leaf or bibb, Rómaine or Cos, and red-leaf)

Sea vegetables (agar agar flakes, sea palm fronds)

Snow peas

Sprouts (alfalfa, chickpea, lentil, mung, radish, aduki, sunflower)

Squash (yellow or crookneck, Italian or zucchini, patty pan or scallop)

Strawberries

Tomatoes

Spring Beans

Fava beans

Green split-pea

Lentils

Spring Grains

Amaranth

Amaranth flakes

Amaranth pasta

Soba (buckwheat noodles)

Whole-grain cold cereals

Special Spring Oil

Almond

Proteins

Eggs

Fish

Lamb

Poultry
Tofu
Tempeh

Dairy
Butter
Goat cheese (feta)
Non- or lowfat cheese
Nonfat yogurt

Dairy Substitute
Soy milk

Spices *(make sure label states "nonirradiated")*
Cilantro
Cinnamon
Coriander
Cumin
Ginger
Marjoram
Thyme

Condiments
Apple cider vinegar
Balsamic vinegar
Barley malt
Brown rice vinegar
Canola mayonnaise
Dijon mustard
Light miso
Raw honey
Rice vinegar
Sesame seeds
Sherry vinegar

Tahini
Tamari

Miscellaneous
Apple juice concentrate
Caffix
Concord grape juice
Kuzu

Spring Diet Menu Sampler

(One-Week Menu Plan)

Monday

Breakfast: Amaranth flakes or whole-grain cold cereal

Nonfat milk

Lunch: Spring Minestrone*

Whole-grain breadsticks

Nonfat cottage cheese

Dinner: Red-Velvet Borscht*

Tarragon roasted chicken

Baby spinach salad

Vinaigrette of sesame seed oil, roasted shallots, oregano, balsamic vinegar, and fresh lemon juice

Tuesday

Breakfast: Bircher muesli (Swiss cold cereal, brand name: Familia) or bran flakes

Nonfat yogurt

Lunch: Turkey cutlet

Sweet peas

Mixed spring green salad with radish and bean sprouts

Dressing of almond oil, fresh lemon juice, chives and salt

Dinner: Warm Asparagus Bisque*

Sweet and Sour Tempeh* over quinoa

---

*Recipe follows.

Wednesday
Breakfast: Poached egg
Whole-grain toast
Lunch: Orient Express Salad*
Dinner: Fish en papillotte or grilled with mushrooms, basil, zucchini, parsley, and fresh lemon juice
Baby vegetable mélange of new potatoes, asparagus tips, baby carrots, green beans, drizzled with fresh flax oil

Thursday
Breakfast: Unsweetened granola
Nonfat yogurt
Lunch: Lentil salad with parsley and chives
Dressing of olive oil, fresh lemon juice, and tamari or low-sodium soy sauce
Whole-grain bread
Dinner: Steamed baby artichokes
Dilled Tofu Mustard*
Charcoal-grilled spring lamb
Oven-roasted new potatoes with fresh thyme and marjoram
Spring greens
Vinaigrette of almond oil, balsamic vinegar, fresh basil, and fresh lemon juice

Friday
Breakfast: Magic Muffins*
Apple butter

---

*Recipe follows.

Lunch:	Quinoa or bulgur with vegetables and sprouts
	Vinaigrette of walnut oil and apple cider vinegar
	Moroccan Carrot Salad*
	Light Miso Tahini Dressing
Dinner:	Garden Rose Soup*
	Grilled salmon steak with leeks, spring onions, and fresh lemon juice
	Blanched beet tops with apple cider vinegar
	Strawberry Delight*

Saturday

Breakfast:	Puffed rice
	Nonfat yogurt
Lunch:	Vichyssoise Bouquet*
	Arugula and radicchio salad with baked goat cheese and whole-grain croutons
	Vinaigrette of olive oil, sherry vinegar, tarragon, and salt
Dinner:	Curried Carrot Soup*
	Roast beef marinated in red wine with thyme and marjoram
	Toasted baby carrots, new baby potatoes, and zucchini
	Mocha Mousse*

Sunday

Brunch:	Huevos rancheros
	Corn tortillas

---

*Recipe follows.

Mixed salad of Romaine lettuce, mushrooms, and alfalfa sprouts with toasted sunflower seeds, fresh chives, and blossoms

Dressing of canola oil, fresh lemon juice, oregano, and salt

Dinner: Amaranth Pasta with Mushroom Lentil Sauce*

Belgian endive

Vinaigrette of almond oil, balsamic vinegar, and anchovy paste

Poached Apples in Grape Juice*

----

*Recipe follows.

Spring Recipes

Spring Minestrone (serves 6)

1 onion, sliced
1 tsp. canola oil
1½ quarts water
2 celery stalks, chopped
3 medium carrots, cut into rounds
1 cup broccoli flowerettes
1 medium potato, cut into cubes
1 cup mushrooms, sliced
1 cup green beans, cut into 1-in. pieces
1 cup sweet peas
1 tsp. fresh margoram
1 tsp. fresh thyme
2 tbsp. fresh chopped parsley
1 strip kombu (sea vegetable), optional
¼ tsp. salt, optional

Sauté onion in oil over low heat until translucent. Add water and bring to a boil. Add all other vegetables and herbs, and stir for 1 minute. Cover and simmer for 20 to 30 minutes (remove kombu). Season with salt, if desired. Soup can be served either hot or cold.

Red-Velvet Borscht (serves 6)

6 large whole beets, scrubbed and rinsed
3 large whole carrots, scrubbed and rinsed
8 cups water
1½ tbsp. light miso

Place beets and carrots in water and bring to a boil. When beets and carrots are soft, remove from water and cut into pieces. Place vegetables and liquid in a blender or food processor and add miso. Blend until smooth, then chill.

Warm Asparagus Bisque (serves 6)

Any vegetable such as mushrooms, carrots, broccoli, or spinach can be substituted for asparagus.

3 cups rolled oats
12 cups water
3 cups asparagus, cut into ½-in. pieces
4 tbsp. light miso
6 sprigs parsley for garnish

Cook oats in water until very soft (about 30 minutes). Add asparagus and cook 10 minutes longer. Add miso and puree in blender or food processor. Garnish with parsley.

Sweet and Sour Tempeh (serves 6)

$\frac{1}{4}$ cup water
$\frac{1}{4}$ cup low-sodium tamari or soy sauce
$\frac{1}{2}$ tsp. ground coriander
1 garlic clove, minced
2 packages tempeh, cut into 1-in. cubes
$\frac{1}{4}$ cup arrowroot

Preheat oven to 350°F. Mix water, tamari, coriander, and garlic. Dip tempeh into mix, then drain and coat with arrowroot. Bake for 20 minutes.

Sweet and Sour Sauce

1 onion, finely chopped
1 tbsp. toasted sesame oil
$1\frac{1}{4}$ cups water
$2\frac{1}{2}$ tbsp. barley malt (or rice malt)
4 tbsp. low-sodium tamari (or soy sauce)
1 tbsp. rice vinegar
1 tbsp. tahini
$\frac{1}{2}$ tsp. fresh grated ginger
2 scallions, finely chopped
2 tsp. kuzu diluted in 2 tbsp. cold water

Sauté onion in oil for 5 minutes. Add water, malt, tamari, vinegar, tahini, ginger, and scallions. Bring to a boil. Thicken with kuzu and serve over tempeh.

Orient Express Salad (serves 6)

> 1 package soba noodles (buckwheat noodles)
> 2 quarts water
> 1 package sea palm fronds (optional)
> 1 package marinated baked tofu, cut into thin strips
> 1 cup grated carrots
> 1 cup scallions, finely chopped
> 1 cup cooked red cabbage
> $\frac{1}{2}$ cup slivered almonds
> $\frac{1}{2}$ cup fresh minced cilantro
> 3 tbsp. almond oil
> 3 tbsp. brown rice vinegar
> $\frac{1}{4}$ tsp. salt (optional)

Boil noodles in water. Drain and set aside. (If using sea palm fronds, cook by first washing, soaking, and boiling till soft. Add to noodles.) Add carrots, tofu, scallions, cabbage, almonds, and, cilantro to noodles and toss. Drizzle with oil, vinegar, and salt. Serve either warm or chilled.

Light Miso Tahini Dressing (serves 6)

> 3 tbsp. tahini
> $1\frac{1}{2}$ tbsp. light miso
> $1\frac{1}{2}$ tbsp. brown rice vinegar
> $\frac{1}{4}$ tsp. barley malt
> $\frac{1}{2}$ tsp. toasted sesame oil
> 4 tbsp. water

Blend all ingredients well. Add more water for a more liquid dressing if desired. This dressing also goes well on steamed greens, broccoli, and cauliflower.

Dilled Tofu Mustard (makes about 1 cup)

    1 8-oz. tofu cake
    2 tbsp. fresh lemon juice
    2 tbsp. Dijon mustard
    2 tbsp. walnut oil or sesame oil
    2 tbsp. fresh minced dill weed
    $\frac{1}{2}$ tsp. salt (optional)

Combine all ingredients in a blender or food processor and puree until creamy. This makes a great dipping sauce for the artichoke and can be used as a tasty dip with raw veggies.

Magic Muffins (serves 8)

    2 tsp. butter
    1 cup plus 2 tbsp. oat bran
    $1\frac{1}{2}$ tsp. baking powder
    1 tsp. ground cinnamon
    $\frac{1}{4}$ tsp. salt (optional)
    1 tbsp. chopped almonds
    $\frac{1}{4}$ cup plus 2 tbsp. nonfat milk
    1 egg, beaten
    2 tbsp. honey
    1 apple, cored and chopped

Preheat oven to 425°F. Butter 8 muffin cups. Mix oat bran, baking powder, cinnamon, and salt in a bowl. Stir in almonds. In a separate bowl combine milk, egg, honey, and chopped apple. Make a well in dry ingredients and add milk mixture. Stir just until moistened. Spoon into prepared muffin cups. Bake for 15 minutes. (Recipe excerpted from Gittleman, A.L.: *Beyond Pritikin*. Bantam, New York, 1988, with permission.)

Moroccan Carrot Salad (serves 6)

　　1 lb. whole carrots, scrubbed and rinsed
　　1 quart water
　　1 garlic clove, peeled
　　$\frac{1}{2}$ tsp. salt (optional)
　　$\frac{1}{2}$ tsp. paprika
　　$\frac{1}{4}$ tsp. ground cumin
　　$\frac{1}{8}$ tsp. cinnamon
　　$\frac{1}{4}$ cup fresh lemon juice
　　2 tbsp. almond oil
　　1 tbsp. chopped parsley for garnish

In a medium saucepan place carrots and garlic in water. Bring to a boil and simmer for about 20 minutes. Discard garlic. Cut carrots into rounds. Combine salt, paprika, cumin, cinnamon, and lemon juice with oil. Blend well and toss with carrots. Garnish with parsley.

Mocha Mousse (serves 4)

　　4 cups apple juice
　　4 tbsp. agar agar flakes or 1 package gelatin
　　4 tbsp. Caffix (instant grain beverage)
　　1 tsp. vanilla extract
　　2 tbsp. tahini

Bring apple juice and agar agar or gelatin to a boil in a medium saucepan. Cover and simmer until agar agar or gelatin is dissolved. Add Caffix and vanilla extract, stirring well. Remove from heat and cool. Let set in refrigerator about 30 to 40 minutes. Blend in tahini until smooth and pour into individual dessert cups.

Garden Rose Soup (serves 6)

    3 heads fresh garlic, peeled
    1 cup canola oil
    1 tbsp. fresh chopped thyme
    1½ quart vegetable stock
    ½ tsp. salt (optional)
    ⅛ tsp. cayenne
    2 tbsp. chopped fresh parsley for garnish

In a heavy bottomed pan sauté garlic in oil over low heat for 20 minutes. Add thyme after 10 minutes. Pour off all but 2 tbsp. of the oil. Add vegetable stock. Cook over low heat for 20 minutes more. Strain and discard garlic. Season with salt and cayenne. Garnish with parsley.

Vichyssoise Bouquet (serves 6)

    2 tsp. extra virgin olive oil
    1 onion, finely chopped
    3 leeks, coarsely chopped
    2 cups rolled oats
    1 bay leaf
    1 sprig fresh thyme
    3½ cups chicken stock
    ¼ tsp. salt (optional)

In heavy saucepan, heat oil and sauté onion and leeks until translucent. Cook oats with bay leaf and thyme in chicken stock until very soft, for about 30 minutes. Discard bay leaf. Puree oats with vegetables until smooth. Add salt, and garnish with scallions.

Strawberry Delight (serves 6)

    3 cups nonfat milk or soy milk
    2¼ cups fresh strawberries
    ¼ cup maple syrup
    ¼ tsp. salt (optional)
    3 level tbsp. agar agar flakes
      or 1 package gelatin
    3 level tsp. kuzu diluted in 3 tbsp. cold water
      or 3 tsp. arrowroot
    ¾ tsp. vanilla extract
    6 strawberries sliced for garnish
    6 sprigs fresh mint for garnish

In a blender or food processor, blend milk and berries until smooth. Combine in a saucepan with maple syrup and salt. Sprinkle in agar agar flakes or gelatin and simmer 1 to 2 minutes, stirring occasionally. Add kuzu or arrowroot to pot while stirring. Remove from heat. Add vanilla extract. Divide into dessert cups and chill for 2 hours. Just before serving, garnish with slices of strawberries and a sprig of fresh mint.

Poached Apples in Grape Juice (serves 6)

    4 cups Concord grape juice
    6 apples
    4 tbsp. kuzu or arrowroot
    4 sprigs fresh mint for garnish

Pour juice into bottom of large pot. Place apples in juice. Cover and simmer until apples are soft but not mushy. Remove apples from juice. Add kuzu or arrowroot to juice and stir until thickened. Pour juice over apples and garnish with mint.

Curried Carrot Soup (serves 6)

2 tsp. extra virgin olive oil
1 onion, coarsely chopped
5 medium carrots, coarsely chopped
1 tsp. thyme
1 tbsp. curry powder
6 cups stock, chicken, or vegetable
2 tbsp. fresh lemon juice
1½ tbsp. light miso
6 sprigs parsley for garnish

Heat oil in saucepan and gently sauté onion until translucent. Add carrots and thyme. Stir in curry powder and sauté a few minutes longer. Add stock and lemon juice. Simmer for 30 to 40 minutes. Blend with miso and garnish with parsley.

Amaranth Pasta with Mushroom Lentil Sauce (serves 6)

1 garlic clove, minced
½ onion, finely chopped
1 stalk celery, finely chopped
1 carrot, finely chopped
2 tbsp. extra virgin olive oil
1½ lb. whole peeled tomatoes (fresh or canned)
1 cup lentils, cooked and drained
1 cup mushrooms, coarsely sliced
¼ tsp. salt (optional)
1 lb. amaranth pasta or whole-grain pasta, cooked and drained

Sauté garlic, onion, celery, and carrots in oil. Add tomatoes and simmer for 20 minutes. Add mushrooms and lentils. Simmer 20 minutes longer. Add salt. Toss with cooked pasta.

Summer Diet

(Mid-June to Mid-September)

Herbs and Spices of Summer
Rosemary, cardamom, savory, mint,
tumeric

Herb Teas for Summer
Lemon grass, red zinger, rose hips,
hibiscus

Shopping List

Summer Produce
Apricots
Avocados
Bananas
Blackberries
Cabbage (red, green, Chinese, or bok choy)
Carrots
Cherries
Corn
Cucumbers
Garlic
Grapefruit
Grapes
Greens (kale, collard, dandelion, mustard, turnip, spinach, Swiss chard, turnip greens, watercress)
Honeydew melon
Kiwi fruit
Jicama
Lemons
Limes

Mangos
Nectarines
New potatoes
Okra
Onions (green, Bermuda, scallions, leeks,
    shallots, chives)
Oranges
Peas
Peaches
Pineapple
Plums
Raspberries
Sea vegetables (arame, agar agar)
Watermelon
Zucchini

Summer Beans
Garbanzos (chickpeas)
Red lentils

Summer Grains
Bulgur wheat
Puffed millet
Yellow corn

Special Summer Oil
Avocado

Proteins
Eggs
Lean beef
Poultry
Shellfish
Tofu

Dairy
Goat cheese (feta)
Non- or lowfat cheese
Nonfat yogurt

Dairy Substitute
Soy milk

Spices (*make sure label states "nonirradiated"*)
Basil
Cayenne pepper
Dill
Marjoram
Mint
Onion powder
Oregano
Paprika
Tarragon
Thyme

Condiments
Apple cider vinegar
Balsamic vinegar
Canola mayonnaise
Capers
Dijon mustard
Light miso
Maple syrup
Nuts (cashews)
Pumpkin seeds
Rice vinegar
Sesame seeds
Sherry vinegar

Tahini
Tamari
Vanilla extract

Miscellaneous
Kuzu

Summer Diet Menu Sampler

(One-Week Menu Plan)

Monday

Breakfast: Mixed cantaloupe and honeydew melon
Nonfat yogurt with fresh mint

Lunch: Tabouleh Salad*
Grated beets with fresh lemon juice

Dinner: Chilled Lemon Miso Soup*
Blackened Red Snapper*
Blanched collard and mustard greens with apple cider vinegar

Tuesday

Breakfast: Papaya
Nonfat yogurt with cardamom

Lunch: Cucumber Dill Soup*
Salade Niçoise with tuna, olives, green beans, tomatoes, and red potatoes on Romaine lettuce

Dinner: Tofu Ceviche*
Corn on the cob, drizzled with flax oil
Steamed kale with savory and apple cider vinegar
Onion Sorbet*

Wednesday

Breakfast: Kiwi and berries
Nonfat yogurt

---

*Recipe follows.

186

Lunch: Crab salad in avocado halves with lime juice

               Molded Vegetable Gel*

Dinner: Charcoal-broiled Cornish game hens with pureed summer squash

               Tossed green salad

               Dressing of sesame oil, fresh lemon juice, and tumeric

Thursday

Breakfast: Fresh fruit medley

               Nonfat yogurt with fresh mint

Lunch: Curried turkey salad with canola mayonnaise, capers, olives, and scallions

               Cucumber salad with nonfat yogurt and chopped dill weed

Dinner: Cream of Watercress Soup*

               Brown Rice with Parsley Nut Sauce*

               Steamed chard and turnip tops with toasted pumpkin seeds and apple cider vinegar

Friday

Breakfast: Puffed millet

               Nonfat milk

Lunch: Celestial Summer Soup*

               Greek salad with feta cheese, red onions, tomatoes, cucumbers, and black olives

               Dressing of olive oil and a touch of salt and pepper

---

*Recipe follows.

Dinner: Vegetable soup with lemon grass
Poached salmon
Baby carrots, sweet peas, and green
  beans with roasted shallots, savory,
  drop of flax oil, and basil
Mango Surprise*

Saturday
Breakfast: Juicy Fruit Soup*
Lunch: Whole-grain short pasta with garban-
  zo beans, fresh thyme, marjoram,
  extra virgin olive oil, and tamari
Dinner: Warm spinach salad
Vinaigrette of balsamic vinegar, ca-
  nola oil, and dijon mustard
Filet mignon with garlic and rose-
  mary
Peach Crisp*

Sunday
Brunch: Herbed omelette with rosemary and
  savory
Summer Confetti Salad*
Dinner: Grilled polenta with pesto and chick-
  peas
Steamed summer vegetable potpourri
Lemon Mousse*

---

*Recipe follows.

Summer Recipes

Tabouleh Salad (serves 6)

 1 cup fresh parsley, finely chopped
 1 stalk celery, finely chopped
 $\frac{1}{2}$ cup capers
 $\frac{1}{2}$ cup scallions, finely chopped
 2 garlic cloves, minced
 $\frac{1}{2}$ cup fresh basil, finely chopped
 5 cups bulgur, cooked
 3 tbsp. fresh lemon juice
 3 tbsp. olive oil
 $1\frac{1}{2}$ tbsp. low-sodium tamari or soy sauce
 $\frac{1}{8}$ tsp. cayenne
 6 leaves fresh mint, finely chopped for garnish

Combine vegetables in bowl. Add bulgur. Blend lemon juice, oil, tamari, and cayenne. Toss with grain and vegetables. Marinate for 30 minutes. Serve chilled garnished with parsley.

Summer Confetti Salad (serves 6)

 10 Belgian endive leaves
 1 avocado, cubed
 1 cup cooked corn
 1 cup grated nonfat cheese
 Juice of 1 lemon
 3 tbsp. avocado oil or sesame oil

Combine all ingredients in salad bowl. Drizzle with dressing of lemon juice and salt.

Chilled Lemon Miso Soup (serves 6)

- $6\frac{1}{2}$ cups chicken or fish stock
- $2\frac{1}{2}$ tbsp. light miso
- 3 tbsp. fresh lemon juice
- 1 medium carrot, cut into flowers
- 3 scallions, finely chopped
- 6 fresh parsley sprigs for garnish

Heat stock in soup pot. Take out 1 cup and dissolve miso in it. Remove pot from heat and add miso, lemon juice, carrot flowers, and scallions. Chill and garnish with parsley.

Blackened Red Snapper (serves 6)

- 1 tbsp. paprika
- $\frac{1}{2}$ tsp. onion powder
- 1 tsp. cayenne
- $\frac{1}{2}$ tsp. dried thyme
- $\frac{1}{2}$ tsp. dried oregano
- $\frac{1}{2}$ tsp. dried basil
- $\frac{1}{2}$ tsp. salt (optional)
- 6 5-oz. red snapper fillets, about 1 in. thick
- 5 tbsp. canola oil
- 6 fresh lemon wedges for garnish

Combine spices on a platter. Place a cast-iron skillet over flame until very hot. Dip red snapper in oil and coat with spice mixture. Place fish in hot skillet for 1 minute. Turn and char other side. Remove from pan. Serve with lemon wedge garnish.

Cucumber Dill Soup (serves 6)

6 cucumbers, peeled and cut into 1½-in. slices
4 cups water
3 tbsp. fresh dill weed, minced
2 tbsp. grated fresh lemon zest
1 tbsp. light miso
Juice of 1 fresh lemon
6 sprigs dill weed for garnish
6 fresh lemon slices for garnish

Place cucumbers in soup pot with water, dill weed, and lemon rind. Cover and simmer until cucumbers are soft. Puree in blender or food processor with miso and lemon juice. Garnish with sprigs of dill weed and lemon slices.

Tofu Ceviche (serves 4)

Juice of 6 fresh limes
½ tsp. salt (optional)
½ lb. tofu, cut into 1-in. slices
1 cup cherry tomatoes (optional)
2 onions, thinly sliced
1 garlic clove, minced
3 tbsp. fresh minced parsley
3 tbsp. fresh minced cilantro
2 avocados, halved

Mix lime juice, garlic, parsley, cilantro, and salt. Pour over tofu slices and marinate for a half hour or more. Pour off excess juice, add tomatoes and onions. Mix and serve in avocado halves.

Onion Sorbet (serves 4)

    2 onions, finely chopped
    1 scallion, finely chopped
    1 tbsp. maple syrup
    2 tbsp. rice vinegar
    $\frac{1}{8}$ tsp. tarragon
    $\frac{1}{8}$ tsp. white pepper
    $\frac{1}{2}$ cup nonfat yogurt

Steam onions until soft and puree in blender or food processor. Mix puree with scallion, maple syrup, tarragon, and pepper. Place in glass bowl and freeze until firm. Blend again until fluffy. Stir in yogurt. Freeze again. This makes a very unusual dessert, and will have your guests raving.

Molded Vegetable Gel (serves 4)

    6 cups chicken or fish stock
    5 tbsp. agar agar flakes or 1 package gelatin
    $\frac{1}{2}$ tsp. salt (optional)
    1 carrot, cut into $\frac{1}{2}$-in. slices
    4 sprigs watercress
    1 zucchini, cut into $\frac{1}{2}$-in. slices
    1 cup arame, soaked in water for 15 minutes
    (optional)

Bring stock to a boil in soup pot. Sprinkle in agar agar flakes or gelatin and salt. Simmer until agar agar or gelatin is dissolved, about 8 to 10 minutes. Arrange vegetables in a shallow glass or Pyrex pan. Carefully pour liquid over vegetables. Let set and serve chilled.

Cream of Watercress Soup (serves 4)

    3 cups vegetable stock
    4 cups fresh watercress, coarsely chopped
    1 tbsp. light miso
    $\frac{1}{2}$ cup nonfat yogurt
    2 scallions, finely chopped for garnish

Place stock in soup pot and bring to a boil. Add watercress and remove from heat. Dissolve miso in 1 cup of soup stock, then return to soup. Blend with yogurt and garnish with scallions.

Brown Rice with Parsley Nut Sauce (serves 6)

    1 cup water
    1 tbsp. canola oil
    1 tbsp. kuzu dissolved in 2 tbsp. water
        or 1 tbsp. arrowroot
    6 scallions, chopped
    1 cup fresh parsley, finely chopped
    $\frac{1}{2}$ cup toasted, chopped cashew pieces
    1 tbsp. tamari
    4 cups brown rice, cooked and fluffed with fork

In medium saucepan, heat water and oil over low heat. Add kuzu or arrowroot and stir until thick. Add scallions, parsley, tamari, and nuts. Serve over rice.

Celestial Summer Soup (serves 6)

1 tbsp. avocado oil or sesame oil
3 leeks, chopped
2 garlic cloves, minced
3 tomatoes, peeled and chopped
5 cups vegetable stock
1 tbsp. light miso
6 sprigs fresh basil for garnish

Heat oil in soup pot. Sauté leeks and garlic until leeks are translucent. Add tomatoes and sauté a few minutes longer. Add stock and simmer 5 minutes. Puree in blender or food processor with basil and miso. Garnish with sprigs of basil. Serve chilled.

Mango Surprise (serves 4)

$1\frac{1}{2}$ cups water
1 tbsp. apple juice concentrate
3 tbsp. agar agar flakes or 1 package gelatin
$1\frac{1}{2}$ cups mango pieces
2 tsp. fresh lime juice

Bring water and apple concentrate to a boil in a small saucepan. Add agar agar flakes or gelatin and simmer until dissolved, about 8 to 10 minutes. Let cool. Puree mango and lime juice in blender or food processor. Add to cooled agar/gelatin mixture and blend until smooth. Divide into serving cups and chill.

Juicy Fruit Soup (serves 6)

- 6 ripe peaches, peeled, pitted, and cubed
- 6 tbsp. fresh lemon juice
- 1 medium cantaloupe, peeled, seeded, and cubed
- 1 cup fresh orange juice
- 1 tsp. vanilla extract
- 1 cup raspberries

Place peaches in heavy saucepan with lemon juice. Simmer for 5 minutes. Remove from heat. Cover and let sit for another 5 minutes. Cool. Puree until creamy. Puree cantaloupe with orange juice until smooth. Add to peach puree. Add vanilla extract and raspberries. Chill.

Peach Crisp (serves 6)

- 4 cups peaches, peeled, pitted, and chopped
- 1 tsp. vanilla extract
- 1 tsp. fresh lemon zest
- 3 tbsp. arrowroot or cornstarch
- 3 cups unsweetened organic apple juice
- 6 cups natural granola with nuts

Preheat oven to 350°F. Mix peaches, vanilla extract, and lemon zest in bowl. Toss lightly with arrowroot. Place in glass baking dish and pour apple juice over mixture. Top with granola. Cover and bake 1 hour.

Lemon Mousse (serves 6)

    6 cups unsweetened organic apple juice
    6 tbsp. agar agar flakes
    Juice of 1 lemon
    1 tsp. vanilla extract
    3 tbsp. tahini
    6 lemon slices for garnish
    6 strands of lemon zest for garnish

In a small saucepan, combine apple juice and agar agar. Bring to a boil. Simmer until agar agar is dissolved, about 8 to 10 minutes. Add lemon juice and vanilla extract. Remove from heat and let set. Blend with tahini until smooth. Pour into individual serving cups. Garnish with lemon slices and zest. (Recipe excerpted from Gittleman, A. L.: *Supernutrition for Women*. Bantam, New York, 1991, with permission.)

Autumn Diet

(Mid-September to Mid-December)

Herbs and Spices of Autumn
Cinnamon, cloves, allspice, nutmeg

Herb Teas for Autumn
Oat straw, slippery elm, flax seed

Shopping List

Autumn Produce
Apples (Golden Delicious, Red Delicious, Cortland, Gravenstein, Jonathan, MacIntosh)
Beets
Cabbage (red, green, Chinese, or bok choy)
Cauliflower
Celery
Cranberries
Fennel
Figs
Grapes
Lettuce
Melons
Mushrooms (wild)
Onions (green, scallions, leeks, shallots, chives)
Parsley
Pears
Persimmon
Pomegranate

Pumpkin

Root vegetables (burdock or gobo, carrots, turnips, parsnips, Daikon radish, celeriac or celery root, Jerusalem artichoke or sunchokes)

Winter squash (acorn, butternut, banana, hubbard, spaghetti)

Autumn Beans

Kidney

Navy (or white or Great Northern)

Soy (in the form of tempeh and tofu)

Autumn Grains

Barley

Cornmeal

Oats

Special Autumn Oil

Sesame (toasted and untoasted)

Proteins

Beef

Eggs

Lamb

Turkey

Dairy

Goat cheese (feta)

Non- or lowfat cheese

Nonfat yogurt

Dairy Substitute

Soy milk

Spices *(make sure label states "nonirradiated")*

Basil
Cardamom
Cilantro
Cinnamon
Clove
Coriander
Cumin
Nutmeg
Oregano

Condiments

Apple cider vinegar
Balsamic vinegar
Canola mayonnaise
Dark miso
Fresh ginger
Maple syrup
Nuts (almonds, walnuts, pistachios)
Pumpkin seeds
Rice vinegar
Sesame seeds
Tahini
Tamari

Miscellaneous

Anchovy paste
Kuzu
Rose water

Autumn Diet Menu Sampler

(One-Week Menu Plan)

Monday

Breakfast: Oatmeal
Nonfat milk

Lunch: Quiche Orientale*
Grated beets with toasted sesame oil and apple cider vinegar

Dinner: Cheezy Onion Soup*
Broiled fillet of sea bass with drop of tamari and fresh grated ginger
Potpourri of lightly steamed seasonal vegetables

Tuesday

Breakfast: Stewed apples with cinnamon and raisins (thickened with arrowroot or kuzu)

Lunch: Broiled natural beef burger
Braised carrots and parsnips with allspice, drizzled with fresh flax oil
Brown rice

Dinner: Artichoke Pasta with Caper Sauce*
Radish and watercress salad
Dressing of sesame oil, fresh lemon juice, and tamari

Wednesday

Breakfast: Seven-grain cereal
Nonfat milk

---

*Recipe follows.

Lunch:	Autumn Harvest Soup*
	Bok choy sautéed in toasted sesame oil and tamari
Dinner:	Heady Tempeh Bourguignon* over steamed barley
	Grated daikon or radish, carrot, and onion salad
	Light Miso Tahini Dressing (see recipe on page 176)
	Yogurt Supreme*

Thursday

Breakfast:	Soft-cooked eggs
	Magic Muffin (see recipe on page 177)
Lunch:	Bean Florentine Soup*
	Celery root salad
	Dressing of canola and fresh lemon juice
Dinner:	Broiled halibut
	Braised Brussels sprouts with pearl onions and nutmeg
	Baked sweet potato

Friday

Breakfast:	Corn meal
	Nonfat milk
Lunch:	Tuna-fish casserole
	Baked broccoli
Dinner:	Mung Bean Dahl*
	Basmati or brown rice
	Spicy Spinach Sauté*

---

*Recipe follows.

Saturday
Breakfast: Barley with freshly grated nutmeg
Nonfat milk
Lunch: Breast of chicken sautéed in toasted sesame oil and garlic
Jerusalem artichoke salad with grated carrots, celery, parsley, and canola mayonnaise
Dinner: Butternut Bisque*
Hearty Hungarian Goulash*
Mixed green salad
Vinaigrette of canola oil, balsamic vinegar, and touch of salt
Persimmon Flan*

Sunday
Brunch: Scrambled eggs
Magic Muffin
(see recipe on page 177)
Steamed cauliflower and leeks
Walnut Miso Sauce*
Dinner: Cream of broccoli soup
Roasted rack of lamb with carrots, turnips, celery, and anise seeds
Company Carrot Cake*

---

*Recipe follows.

Autumn Recipes

Quiche Orientale (serves 6 to 8)

   Crust: 1 cup whole wheat pastry flour
        $\frac{1}{4}$ cup sesame oil
        1 tbsp. rice vinegar
        $\frac{1}{4}$ tsp. salt (optional)
        $\frac{1}{2}$ cup water

Place flour, oil, vinegar, and salt into a food processor or blender. Slowly add water while machine is running until mixture forms a ball. Press into oiled pie dish.

   Filling: 2 lbs. tofu
        1 tbsp. tahini
        1 tsp. fresh grated ginger
        1 tbsp. low-sodium tamari or soy sauce
        $3\frac{1}{2}$ cups broccoli flowerettes
        $\frac{1}{4}$ cup grated carrot

Preheat oven to 350°F. Break tofu into pieces and place in blender or food processor with tahini, ginger, and tamari. Blend until smooth. Blanch the broccoli flowerettes for a few minutes and set aside. Spoon tofu mixture into unbaked pie crust. Arrange carrot and broccoli, pressing them slightly into the mixture. Cover and bake for 20 minutes. Remove cover and bake another 5 to 10 minutes, or until tofu is slightly brown. Let cool 10 minutes before cutting.

Cheezy Onion Soup (serves 6)

    3 onions, thinly sliced
    2 tbsp. sesame oil
    8 cups fish stock
    ½ tsp. tamari
    1 cup grated non- or lowfat cheese (I suggest
        Lifetime brand Swiss, mozzarella, cheddar, or
        Monterey Jack)
    6 sprigs parsley for garnish

Sauté onions in oil until very soft. Add stock and
simmer 10 minutes. Add tamari and cheese. Garnish
with parsley.

Artichoke Pasta with
Caper Sauce (serves 6)

    3 tbsp. olive oil
    1 garlic clove, minced
    ⅛ tsp. crushed chili pepper
    1½ lb. whole peeled tomatoes (fresh or canned)
    ½ cup capers
    ½ cup chopped black olives
    1½ tsp. anchovy paste
    ¼ tsp. salt (optional)
    1 lb. artichoke pasta, cooked and drained

Heat oil in saucepan over low heat. Sauté garlic and
chili pepper. Add tomatoes, olives, and capers. Simmer uncovered for 20 to 30 minutes. Add anchovy
paste. Toss with pasta and serve.

Autumn Harvest Soup (serves 6)

    3 tbsp. sesame oil
    1 cup chopped onions
    1 cup chopped mushrooms
    3 tbsp. sherry
    8 cups vegetable stock
    $\frac{1}{4}$ cup barley
    $\frac{1}{2}$ tsp. salt (optional)
    6 sprigs fresh parsley for garnish

Heat oil in soup pot and sauté onions until translucent. Add mushrooms and sherry. Sauté a few minutes longer. Add stock, salt, and barley. Simmer for 45 minutes. Garnish with parsley.

Heady Tempeh Bourguignon (serves 6)

    1 tbsp. sesame oil
    2 large onions, sliced
    $\frac{1}{2}$ lb. tempeh, cubed
    2 cups red wine
    1 tbsp. dark miso
    2 cups mushrooms, thinly sliced

Preheat oven to 350°F. Heat oil in skillet and sauté onions until limp and translucent, but not brown. Set aside. Bake tempeh for 15 minutes. Add to skillet. Pour in wine and cook for a few minutes. Remove a few tablespoons of liquid from skillet. Dissolve miso in liquid and return to skillet. Add mushrooms and cook a few more minutes. Serve over steamed barley.

Yogurt Supreme (serves 6)

6 cups nonfat yogurt
½ tsp. cardamom
6 tbsp. maple syrup
Pistachios, toasted and chopped, for garnish

Combine all ingredients into a bowl. Divide into individual serving cups. Garnish with pistachios.

Bean Florentine Soup (serves 6)

2 cups navy beans
1 strip kombu (sea vegetable, optional)
8 cups water
½ cup chopped celery
½ cup chopped onion
1 tbsp. fresh chopped oregano
1 tbsp. fresh chopped basil
1 tsp. garlic, minced
2 cups chopped fresh spinach
¼ tsp. tamari

Place beans (and kombu) in soup pot with water. Cover and cook about 1½ hours until soft and creamy. Add celery, onion, oregano, basil, and garlic. Cook 30 minutes longer. Add spinach and cook 5 more minutes. Add tamari and serve.

Mung Bean Dahl (serves 6)

1 tbsp. sesame oil
½ tsp. cinnamon
½ tsp. cumin
1 minced onion
3 cups mung beans or chickpeas
1 strip kombu
12 cups water
¼ tsp. salt (optional)
6 sprigs fresh cilantro for garnish
6 fresh lemon slices for garnish

Heat oil in soup pot. Sauté cinnamon, cumin, and onion. Add beans, kombu, and water. Cook for 45 to 60 minutes. Add salt. Garnish with cilantro and lemon slices. Serve over basmati or brown rice.

Spicy Spinach Sauté (serves 6)

1 tbsp. sesame oil
1 large onion, sliced
1 tsp. coriander
1 tsp. cumin
1 tsp. ground clove
1 tsp. freshly grated nutmeg
1 tsp. cinnamon
1½ lb. fresh spinach, well rinsed and drained
½ cup nonfat farmer's cheese

Heat oil in skillet over low heat. Sauté onion, coriander, cumin, clove, nutmeg, and cinnamon until onion is translucent. Add spinach and sauté until limp. Remove from heat and crumble in cheese.

Butternut Bisque (serves 6)

1 large butternut squash, skinned and cubed
4 cups water
$\frac{1}{2}$ tsp. salt (optional)
$\frac{1}{4}$ tsp. cumin
$\frac{1}{4}$ tsp. coriander
$\frac{1}{4}$ tsp. fresh grated ginger
$\frac{1}{4}$ tsp. garlic powder
4 sprigs fresh parsley for garnish
12 toasted almonds for garnish
6 heaping tbsp. nonfat yogurt

Place water and squash in soup pot. Cover and simmer for 5 minutes. Add salt and cumin, coriander, ginger, and garlic. Continue simmering for 15 minutes. Puree in blender or food processor. Serve garnished with sprig of parsley, chopped toasted almonds, and a dollop of yogurt.

Hearty Hungarian Goulash (serves 6)

3 tbsp. canola oil
1 cup onion, sliced
$2\frac{1}{2}$ lb. beef, cut into 2-in. strips
1 tsp. paprika
$\frac{1}{4}$ tsp. salt (optional)
$\frac{1}{2}$ cup dry white wine
1 lb. whole peeled tomatoes (fresh or canned)

Preheat oven to 350°F. Heat canola oil in large skillet over medium heat. Sauté onion and meat. When onions are golden, add paprika and salt. Add wine and cook a few minutes longer. Add tomatoes. Cover and bake for $1\frac{1}{2}$ hours. Check after 45 minutes and add more water if necessary.

Company Carrot Cake (serves 6)

    5 cups whole-wheat pastry flour
    2 tbsp. baking powder
    1 tsp. cinnamon
    4 cups unsweetened apple juice
    2 tbsp. canola oil
    1 tsp. vanilla extract
    ½ cup water
    1 tbsp. grated orange zest
    1 cup grated carrot
    1 cup currants
    3 egg whites, whipped
    ¼ tsp. salt

Preheat oven to 350°F. In a large mixing bowl, combine flour, baking powder, and cinnamon. In another bowl, combine apple juice, canola oil, vanilla extract, water, and orange zest. Stir liquid into flour mixture and combine well. Add carrots and currants. Gently fold in egg whites. Add salt. Pour into oiled glass baking dish and bake for 45 minutes. Cool and pour glaze over top.

    Glaze: 3 cups unsweetened apple juice
            2½ cups fresh orange juice
            2 tbsp. maple syrup
            ⅓ cup kuzu dissolved in ½ cup water
              or 1 package gelatin

Bring apple and orange juice to a boil in a saucepan. Add maple syrup and kuzu or gelatin. Stir until thick. Pour over cooled cake.

Persimmon Flan (serves 6)

>   2 tbsp. agar agar flakes or 1 package gelatin
>   ¾ cup water
>   2 cups nonfat or soy milk
>   2 cups pureed persimmon pulp (about 4 to 5
>   large persimmons)
>   ½ cup maple syrup
>   ½ tsp. salt

In medium saucepan, heat agar agar or gelatin in water until dissolved. Add milk and bring to a boil. Mix persimmon, maple syrup, and salt. Pour hot liquid through strainer into puree. Whisk well and pour into 6 individual custard cups. Refrigerate.

Walnut Miso Sauce (makes 1 cup)

>   1 cup chopped walnuts
>   3 tbsp. light miso
>   2 tbsp. rice vinegar
>   2 tbsp. dijon mustard
>   3 tbsp. water

Blend all ingredients in blender or food processor.

Winter Diet

(Mid-December to Mid-March)

Herbs and Spices of Winter
Caraway, anise, ginger, coriander, garlic, saffron

Herb Teas for Winter
Blueberry leaf, raspberry leaf

Shopping List

Winter Produce
Apples (Cortland, Jonathan, MacIntosh, Pippin, Rome Beauty)
Blackberries
Blueberries
Broccoli
Brussels sprouts
Cabbage (red, green, Chinese, or bok choy)
Chicory
Dates, dried
Figs, dried
Garlic
Leeks
Lettuce
Mushrooms (boletu or beefsteak, enoki or straw mushrooms, oyster, shiitake or black forest)
Onions (pearl or boiling)
Parsley
Potatoes

Root vegetables (burdock or gobo, carrots, turnips, parsnips, daikon radish, celeriac or celery root, Jerusalem artichoke or sunchokes)

Sea vegetables (dulse, kombu, nori, hijiki, wakame, sea palm frond)

Winter squash (acorn, butternut, banana, hubbard, spaghetti)

Winter Beans
Aduki
Black
Pinto

Winter Grains
Amaranth flour
Blue corn
Buckwheat flour
Kasha (buckwheat groats)
Rye
Whole-wheat pastry flour

Special Winter Oil
Peanut

Proteins
Beef
Chicken
Eggs
Nuts (peanuts, cashews)

Dairy
Goat cheese (feta)
Non- or lowfat cheese
Nonfat yogurt

Dairy Substitute
Soy milk

Spices *(make sure label states "nonirradiated")*
Bay leaf
Black pepper
Cayenne
Ginger
Oregano
Thyme

Condiments
Apple cider vinegar
Balsamic vinegar
Butterscotch extract
Canola mayonnaise
Dark miso
Dijon mustard
Dried apples
Dried apricots
Maple syrup
Nuts (pecans)
Pumpkin seeds
Raisins
Rice vinegar
Sesame seeds
Tahini
Tamari
Unsweetened coconut flakes
Vanilla extract

Miscellaneous
Aluminum-free baking powder (Royal, Rumford brands)

Toasted wheat germ

Winter Diet Menu Sampler

(One-Week Menu Plan)

Monday

Breakfast: Kasha (buckwheat groats)
                Nonfat milk

Lunch: Golden Squash Soup*
                Overnight Sourdough Bread*

Dinner: Tangy Holiday Chicken*
                Salad of wilted cabbage, daikon or radish, celery
                Vinaigrette of extra virgin olive oil, rice vinegar, and tamari

Tuesday

Breakfast: Scrambled eggs
                Whole-grain toast

Lunch: Winter Bean Pâté*
                Blue corn tortillas

Dinner: Roast beef with wine, carrots, and onions
                Wild and brown rice with beefsteak and shiitake mushrooms
                Braised celery and parsnips with anise seeds

Wednesday

Breakfast: Cream of rye cereal
                Nonfat milk

Lunch: Hijiki Noodles*
                Caesar salad

---

*Recipe follows.

Dinner: Wonderful Winter Stew*
                Cod Parmentier*

Thursday
Breakfast: Truly Fruity Muffins* with a bit of flax
                seed oil or apple butter
Lunch: Ground lean lamb patty
                Burdock Carrot Kimpara*
Dinner: Brazilian Bean Dream*
                Green salad with toasted walnuts
                Vinaigrette of sesame oil and apple
                cider vinegar

Friday
Breakfast: Nine-grain cereal
                Nonfat milk
Lunch: Steamed Jerusalem artichoke hearts
                and assorted root vegetables
                Warm Anchovy Sauce*
Dinner: Spinach Meat Loaf*
                Bok Choy in Ginger and Garlic
                Sauce*
                Bamboo shoots in peanut oil
                German Carob Cake*

Saturday
Breakfast: Soft-cooked eggs
                Rye toast
Lunch: Potato Leek Pie*
                Warm red cabbage and caraway seed
                salad
Dinner: Wilted spinach salad

---

*Recipe follows.

Vinaigrette of canola oil, balsamic
    vinegar, and a dash of salt
Bountiful Bouillabaise*
Pears in Red Wine Sauce*

Sunday
Brunch: Buckwheat Pancakes*
Sautéed mushrooms, garlic, onions,
    and parsley in red wine
Small green salad
Dressing of peanut oil, parsley, and
    lemon juice
Dinner: Miso soup
Seasonal root vegetables
Spiced Beef with Wine*
Pumpkin pie

---

*Recipe follows.

Winter Recipes

Bountiful Bouillabaisse (serves 6)

    4 tbsp. peanut oil
    1 onion, sliced
    2 leeks, chopped
    1 carrot, chopped
    1 stalk celery, chopped
    1 lb. cod fillet, cut into 2-in. pieces
    4 lb. rockfish fillet, cut into 2-in. pieces
    2 garlic cloves, chopped
    1 bay leaf
    1 tsp. fennel seed
    2 tbsp. Pernod (optional)
    $\frac{1}{2}$ cup white wine
    2 medium tomatoes, sliced
    $\frac{1}{2}$ tsp. salt (optional)
    $\frac{1}{2}$ tsp. black pepper
    2 tbsp. fresh minced parsley for garnish

In heavy pan, heat oil and sauté onion, leeks, carrot, and celery. Add fish, garlic, bay leaf, and fennel. Sauté a few minutes more. Add Pernod, wine, and tomatoes. Add water to cover fish and vegetables. Simmer for 30 minutes. Add salt and pepper and serve with parsley garnish.

Brazilian Bean Dream (serves 6)

1 onion, chopped
2 garlic cloves, minced
2 tbsps. canola oil
1 cup dry black beans
2 cups chicken stock
1 cup red wine
1 bay leaf
$\frac{1}{4}$ tsp. pepper
2 celery stalks
1 tomato, chopped
$\frac{1}{4}$ tsp. salt (optional)

In large heavy pot, sauté onion and garlic in oil. Add beans, stock, wine, bay leaf, and pepper. Bring to a boil and simmer 2 minutes. Cover and let sit 1 hour. Add celery and tomato. Simmer for 2 hours until beans are tender. Add salt. Remove 1 cup of beans, mash, and return to pot. Remove bay leaf.

Golden Squash Soup (serves 6)

1 large butternut squash, skinned and cubed
5 cups water
$\frac{1}{4}$ cup fresh lemon juice
$1\frac{1}{2}$ tbsp. light miso
$\frac{1}{2}$ cup chopped parsley for garnish

Place squash in soup pot with water and lemon juice. Cover and simmer for 30 minutes. Remove 1 cup of liquid and dissolve miso in it. Add back to pot. Serve with parsley garnish.

Spinach Meat Loaf (serves 6)

   1 lb. lean ground sirloin
   1 garlic clove, minced
   1 onion, minced
   ½ tsp. dried thyme
   1 egg
   2 egg whites
   ½ cup toasted wheat germ
   ½ tsp. salt (optional)
   ⅛ tsp. pepper
   1 cup cooked chopped spinach

Preheat oven to 350°F. Combine meat, garlic, onion, thyme, egg, egg whites, salt, pepper, and wheat germ. Place half of mixture in oiled baking dish and pat down. Place chopped spinach on top of meat and place other half of meat mixture on top of spinach. Form into a meat-loaf shape. Place on rack set over a pan of water and bake 1 to 1¼ hours.

Bok Choy in Ginger and Garlic Sauce
(serves 6)

   3 bok choy, sliced into 1½-in. strips
   2 tbsp. toasted sesame oil
   2 garlic cloves, minced
   2 tsp. grated fresh ginger
   1 tsp. kuzu, diluted in 1 tbsp. cold water
   ¼ cup low-sodium tamari or soy sauce

Sauté bok choy in oil with garlic and ginger. Add diluted kuzu and stir until thickened. Add tamari.

Wonderful Winter Stew (serves 6)

3 dried shiitake mushrooms, soaked in water 10 minutes and sliced
1 cup water
1 tbsp. peanut oil
1 medium daikon radish, sliced
1 parsnip, diced
$\frac{1}{2}$ cup water
1 tbsp. fresh grated ginger
1 tbsp. kuzu, diluted in 2 tbsp. cold water
2 tbsp. low-sodium tamari or soy sauce
1 scallion, chopped for garnish

Heat oil in heavy skillet over medium heat and sauté daikon. Add parsnip and shiitake mushroom. Stir and reduce heat. Add $\frac{1}{2}$ cup water and simmer for 20 minutes. Add ginger. Add kuzu and stir until thickened. Season with tamari and garnish with scallion.

Hijiki Noodles (serves 6)

1 lb. whole-wheat noodles, cooked and drained
1 package hijiki seaweed, soaked in water, rinsed, and cut into strips
1 cup grated carrots
$\frac{1}{2}$ cup chopped celery
$\frac{1}{2}$ cup fresh minced parsley
$\frac{1}{2}$ cup minced scallions
1 clove garlic, minced
6 tbsp. extra virgin olive oil

Combine all ingredients. Toss with olive oil. Let stand a half hour before serving. (Recipe excerpted from Gittleman, A. L.: *Supernutrition for Women*. Bantam, New York, 1991, with permission.)

Truly Fruity Muffins (makes 20)

4 cups dried unsulphured apricots, soaked
4 cups dried unsulphured apples, soaked
4 cups apple juice concentrate
1 tsp. vanilla extract
7 cups whole-wheat pastry flour
2 tsp. baking powder
2 tbsp. cinnamon
$\frac{1}{8}$ tsp. salt
2 cups raisins
$\frac{1}{4}$ cup canola oil

Preheat oven to 375°F. Butter 20 muffin cups. In medium mixing bowl, combine apricots, apples, apple concentrate, and vanilla extract. In a separate bowl, mix flour, baking powder, cinnamon, and salt. Combine fruit mixture with flour mixture. Add raisins. Spoon into prepared muffin cups and bake for 20 minutes.

Burdock Carrot Kimpira (serves 6)

1 tbsp. canola oil
1 tsp. toasted sesame oil
4 medium carrots, scrubbed and cut into shavings
2 medium burdock roots, scrubbed and cut into shavings
$\frac{1}{2}$ tsp. tamari

Heat canola and sesame oil in heavy skillet. Sauté carrot and burdock for a few minutes. Add tamari. In the Orient, burdock is considered to be very blood building and helpful for women's reproductive organs.

Buckwheat Pancakes (makes 24)

$\frac{1}{2}$ cup buckwheat flour
$\frac{1}{2}$ cup whole-wheat pastry flour
$1\frac{1}{2}$ tsp. baking soda
$1\frac{1}{2}$ tsp. ground cinnamon
$1\frac{1}{2}$ cups warm water
2 tbsp. fresh lemon juice
3 tbsp. canola oil
2 tbsp. maple syrup

In a medium mixing bowl, combine the flour, baking soda, and cinnamon. In a separate small bowl, mix the water, lemon juice, oil, and maple syrup. Combine the liquid with the flour mixture for a thin batter. Drop spoonfuls of batter onto a preheated oiled griddle or frying pan. Cook about 5 minutes on each side, until pancakes are brown on both sides.

Pears in Red Wine Sauce (serves 6)

6 pears, cored, peeled, and halved
8 cups red wine
2 cups unsweetened apple juice
1 stick cinnamon
3 whole cloves
1 tsp. lemon zest
1 tbsp. maple syrup
3 tbsp. kuzu dissolved in 5 tbsp. cold water
    or 1 package gelatin

Place pears in heavy pan and cover with wine, apple juice, cinnamon, cloves, lemon zest, and syrup. Cover and simmer for 30 minutes. Remove pears. Add kuzu or gelatin to remaining liquid and stir until thick. Remove cinnamon and cloves. Pour sauce over pears.

Tangy Holiday Chicken (serves 6)

    3 tbsp. sesame oil
    ½ tsp. grated fresh ginger
    ½ tsp. coriander
    ½ tsp. cardamom
    ½ tsp. cumin
    3 whole chicken breasts, skinned and halved
    1 onion, sliced
    2 carrots, sliced
    1 cup cauliflower flowerettes
    1 cup green beans, cut into 1-in. pieces
    2 cups water
    ¼ tsp. salt (optional)
    1 large butternut squash, cooked and pureed

Heat oil in skillet. Sauté ginger, coriander, cardamom, and cumin in oil. Add chicken, onion, and carrots. Sauté until chicken is golden and onions are translucent. Add cauliflower and beans. Add water and salt. Cover and cook 15 more minutes. Add pureed squash and cook 5 minutes longer.

Winter Bean Pâté (makes 4 cups)

    4 cups aduki beans, cooked and drained
    1 tbsp. light miso
    ¼ tsp. cayenne pepper
    2 tbsp. rice vinegar
    2 tbsp. extra virgin olive oil
    1 garlic clove, minced
    1 tsp. dried thyme
    1 tsp. dried oregano

Blend all ingredients in blender or food processor. Serve with tortillas or crackers.

Cod Parmentier (serves 6)

1 whole 4-lb. cod
6 potatoes, thinly sliced
2 tbsp. peanut oil
$\frac{1}{4}$ tsp. salt (optional)
2 onions, sliced
4 celery stalks, finely chopped
1 bay leaf, chopped
$\frac{1}{4}$ tsp. salt
$\frac{1}{8}$ tsp. pepper
5 tomatoes, sliced
6 sprigs fresh parsley for garnish
6 fresh lemon slices for garnish

Preheat oven to 350°F. In oiled baking dish, spread one layer of potato slices. Drizzle olive oil and salt over potatoes. Place onion slices on top. Stuff fish with mixture of celery, bay leaf, pepper, and salt. Place on top of onions. Place tomato slices around and on top of fish. Cover and bake about 1$\frac{1}{2}$ hours. Garnish with parsley and lemon.

Warm Anchovy Sauce (serves 6)

6 tbsp. extra virgin olive oil
8 anchovy fillets, well rinsed, drained, and chopped
8 garlic cloves, crushed

Heat oil over medium low heat. Remove from heat and add garlic. Let sit for about 10 minutes. Do not cook. Stir anchovies into mixture and keep warm. Use as a sauce over vegetables.

German Carob Cake (makes 1 cake)

2½ cups whole-wheat pastry flour
½ cup carob powder
2 tsp. baking soda
½ tsp. salt
1 cup plus 2 tbsp. water
1 cup plus 2 tbsp. maple syrup
½ cup canola oil
1½ tsp. vanilla extract
1½ tbsp. apple cider vinegar

Preheat oven to 350°F. Butter and flour 3 cake pans.
In a medium mixing bowl, combine flour, carob,
baking soda, and salt. In a separate mixing bowl, mix
water, syrup, oil, vanilla extract, and vinegar. Stir
liquid into flour mixture. Pour into prepared cake
pans and bake for 20 minutes, until toothpick comes
out clean. Frost cake when cool.

Frosting: 1½ cups water
1½ cups maple syrup
½ tsp. salt (optional)
3 tbsp. kuzu dissolved in 5 tbsp. water
or 1 package gelatin
3 tbsp. vanilla extract
½ tsp. butterscotch extract
1½ cups chopped toasted pecans
1½ cups dried coconut flakes

Heat water, maple syrup, and salt in saucepan. Add
kuzu or gelatin and stir into hot mixture. Add vanilla,
butterscotch, pecans, and coconut. Spread between
cake layers and on top of cake when cake is cool but
frosting is still hot.

Overnight Sourdough Bread (makes 1 loaf)

Sourdough starter: 1 cup whole-wheat flour
$\frac{1}{2}$ cup cooked brown rice
2 cups water

In a large ceramic bowl, mix well and cover. Let stand in cool dark place for 3 to 4 days.

Bread: 2 cups sourdough starter
$\frac{1}{2}$ cup canola oil
6 cups whole-wheat flour
1 cup water
$\frac{1}{4}$ tsp. salt

Mix all ingredients together and knead on a floured surface for about 10 minutes until dough is elastic. Place in oven with pilot light on and let stand overnight (approximately 12 hours). Bake in preheated oven at 350°F for 1 hour.

Potato Leek Pie (serves 6)

3 medium potatoes, cut into large cubes
2 large leeks, cut into large slices
2 tsp. dried thyme
$\frac{1}{2}$ tsp. salt (optional)
6 cups vegetable stock
2 tbsp. canola oil
$\frac{1}{2}$ cup fresh parsley, minced
$\frac{1}{2}$ cup whole-wheat bread crumbs

Preheat oven to 350°F. Grease a 9″ × 12″ baking dish with oil. Place potatoes and leeks into soup pot. Add thyme, salt, and stock. Cover and cook over medium heat for 30 minutes. Pour mixture into baking dish and sprinkle parsley and crumbs over top. Bake uncovered for 15 minutes.

Spiced Beef with Wine (serves 6)

- 1 2-lb. fillet, all visible fat removed
- 2 carrots, chopped
- 1 onion, sliced
- 1 celery stalk, chopped
- 2 garlic cloves, minced
- 4 whole cloves
- $\frac{1}{2}$ tsp. salt (optional)
- $\frac{1}{8}$ tsp. pepper
- 3 cups red wine
- 4 tbsp. extra virgin olive oil
- 1 lb. mushrooms
- 1 tbsp. grape-seed oil

Marinate meat with vegetables, garlic, cloves, salt, and pepper in wine for 2 to 3 hours. In heavy pan, heat oil. Remove meat from marinade and brown in oil. Strain remaining marinade, and cook in saucepan over high heat until marinade is reduced to half. Add back to meat. Cover and cook over low heat for 2 hours. In separate skillet, sauté mushrooms in 1 tbsp. grape-seed oil. Remove meat from pan. Slice and place on serving platter. Pour sauce and mushrooms over meat.

Conclusion

Congratulations! By reading this book you have taken the very first step toward understanding a nutritional approach to menopause. You have learned that menopause does not happen overnight. It is the culmination of years of lifestyle habits, both good and bad. You have read how heredity, smoking, diet, exercise and stress all take their toll and contribute to the "change of life."

The good news, however, is that it is *never too late to change your habits*—all it takes is your desire and commitment to take responsibility for your own health. Step by step, one day at a time, you can begin to build, or even rebuild, a sound foundation for a comfortable menopause and quality longevity.

Start simply by cutting back on sugar, coffee, artificial sweeteners and saturated fat. Start adding the good oils to your diet. Use olive oil and canola oil for cooking and baking. Experiment with sesame oil for salad dressings and the heart-healthy flax oil for dribbling onto veggies or whole grains. Avoid margarine and vegetable shortening. For fiber and hard-to-come-by minerals, add more beans and sea vegetables to your menu plans.

Slowly increase your exercise. Begin walking regularly if you aren't currently doing it. Remember that walking, light aerobics, and weight training help to strengthen bone mass. Not only is exercise good for your body, but it is also a great stress reliever.

Most of all, make this a special time of life for *you*. Take some quiet time for yourself on a daily basis. Meditation and deep breathing are excellent tools for calming the mind and smoothing out the ups and downs of modern-day living. Reading uplifting affirmations and spiritual books can often take you outside of yourself and renew your perspective on life. Treat yourself well and listen to your body/mind signals. Menopause can be a wonderful time for taking inventory of all aspects of your life. Explore this time with joy and adventure because, for many women, the best is still ahead.

I hope this book will be as useful to you as researching it has been for me. It is comforting to know that the classic symptoms of menopause—night sweats, vaginal dryness, insomnia and mood swings—are not inevitable. There are many vitamins, herbs, essential fatty acids and homeopathic preparations that can help to balance a changing body chemistry—without side effects. The shopping list and recipe section will help guide you to make the dietary recommendations discussed throughout the book into a delicious and nutritious reality.

Taking control of your menopause now will start you on a journey to continued health, vitality and radiance. May your journey be blessed with happiness and wisdom as well.

Resources

Menopause

North American Menopause Society
Department of Obstetrics/Gynecology
University MacDonald Women's Hospital
2074 Abington Rd.
Cleveland, OH 44106

This organization can refer you to menopause specialists from a listing of over 1,000 gynecologists, orthopedists, and other health-care professionals.

A Friend Indeed Publications, Inc.
P.O. Box 1710
Champlain, NY 12919

Box 515, Place du Parc Station
Montreal, Quebec, Canada H2W 2P1

A Friend Indeed is a monthly newsletter devoted to menopause. It features research updates and readers' experiences on a variety of menopause-related concerns. A one-year subscription (10 issues) is $30.00, payable to *A Friend Indeed*. Canadians should add $2.10, for a total of $32.10. If you would like a listing of topics covered in previous issues, you can send a stamped, addressed envelope.

Menopause News
2074 Union Street
San Francisco, CA 94123
(800) 241-6366

An independent bimonthly newsletter with the latest medical information about menopause as well as psychological perspectives. It covers conventional as well as alternative approaches. *Menopause News* includes book reviews, letters, and first-person accounts. A one-year subscription costs $24 for individuals and $30 for institutions. Back issues are available for $3.50 each on such topics as insomnia, fine-tuning estrogen, breast cancer support, fibroids, and more.

Nutrition

National Women's Health Network
1325 G Street NW
Washington, D.C. 20005

Write to the network for information on a variety of women's health issues.

The Felix Letter
P.O. Box 7094
Berkeley, CA 94707

Berkeley nutritionist Clara Felix publishes this independent health newsletter that specializes in the most current information on fats and oils. One year (6 issues) is $11, while two years (12 issues) is $20. Back issues are available at $4 per issue. Ask for a sample issue plus index.

Dr. Julian Whitaker's *Health and Healing Newsletter*
Phillips Publishing, Inc.
7811 Montrose Rd.
Potomac, MD 20854

This monthly newsletter provides the latest updates on health and healing from Julian Whitaker, M.D., and Jane Heimlich. Subscriptions are $69 per year.

Price-Pottenger Nutrition Foundation
P.O. Box 2614
La Mesa, CA 91943
(619) 582-4168

The Price-Pottenger Nutrition Foundation is a nonprofit, tax-exempt educational organization dedicated to the promotion of enhanced health through an awareness of ecology, lifestyle, and healthy food production for good nutrition. At its core are the landmark works of Drs. Weston A. Price and Francis M. Pottenger, Jr., pioneers in modern nutrition research.

The foundation maintains a list of nutrition-oriented health-care professionals, which can link patients to providers in their area. Memberships begin at $25.00.

Citizens for Health
P.O. Box 368
Tacoma, WA 98401
(206) 922-2457

This consumer-oriented group is dedicated to keeping you informed on the latest government regulations affecting health-care options. Citizens for Health has an immediate FAX network and a quarterly newsletter. Members can join for $20, benefactors for $75, and founders at $250. Each of these rates entitles you to different benefits.

Seeds of Change
621 Old Santa Fe Trail, #10
Santa Fe, NM 87501
(505) 983-8956
FAX: (505) 983-8957

Seeds of Change offers commercial quantities of organic seed to backyard gardeners and retailers nationally. Ask for their award winning *Seeds of Change Catalog*.

Health Harvest Unlimited, Inc.
P.O. Box 427
Fairfax, CA 94930
(415) 924-7445

Health Harvest provides a unique selection of "healthy" gifts, ranging from Sole-Sox to spiritual T-shirts and sweatshirts. Health Harvest also distributes Elson Haas' *Staying Healthy with Nutrition: The Complete Guide to Diet and Nutritional Medicine*. This book is a wonderful resource on many disease conditions and life-cycle ailments. Write for a catalog.

Uni-Key Health Systems
542 Alto St.
Santa Fe, NM 87501
(800) 888-4353

This company has distributed supplements to my own clients and readers for over 3 years. Ask for a brochure of all the latest products. If you can't find my three books *Beyond Pritikin, Supernutrition for Women,* and *Guess What Came to Dinner* in the bookstore, Uni-Key can send them to you directly.

American Academy of Nutrition
3408 Sausalito
Corona del Mar, CA 92625-1638
(800) 290-4226

The American Academy of Nutrition offers nutrition education courses through home study and is the *only* nutrition home-study school in the world that is accredited by the U.S. Department of Education's National Home Study Council. The Academy is also approved as a continuing education provider for many groups, including nurses and the American College of Sports Medicine, and is approved by the

U.S. Department of Defense for military tuition assistance. As Director of Continuing Education for the American Academy of Nutrition, I highly recommend their nutrition courses for anyone who wishes to increase their knowledge in this vital subject.

Notes

1: Menopause

1. Wurtman J: "Weight Gain at Menopause." *A Friend Indeed* 9(4):1–3, 1992

3: The Calcium Craze

1. McCarron DA, Morris CD: "Blood Pressure Response to Oral Calcium in Persons with Mild to Moderate Hypertension: A Randomized Double-Blind Placebo-Controlled Crossover Trial." *Ann Intern Med* 103:825, 1985
2. Johnson NE, Smith EL, Freudenheim JL: "Effects on Blood Pressure of Calcium Supplementation of Women." *Am J Clin Nutr* 42:12, 1985
3. Bierennbaum ML, et al: "The Effect of Dietary Calcium Supplementation on Blood Pressure and Serum Lipid Levels, Preliminary Report." *Nutr Rep Intl* 36:1147, 1987

4. Lakshmanan FL, et al: "Calcium and Phosphorus Intakes, Balances, and Blood Levels of Adults Consuming Self-Selected Diets." *Amer J Clin Nutr* 40:1368, 1984

5. Hollingberg P, Massey L: "Effect of Dietary Caffeine and Sucrose on Urinary Calcium Excretion in Adolescents." *Federal Protocol* 45:375, 1968

6. Coats CD: "Negative Effects of High Protein Diet." *Family Practice Recertification* 12(12): 80–88, 1990

7. Spenser H, et al: "Effects of Small Doses of Aluminum-Containing Antacids on Calcium and Phosphorus Metabolism," *American Journal of Clinical Nutrition* 36:32, 1982

8. Recker RR: "Calcium Absorption and Achlorhydria." *New Engl J Med* 313:70, 1985

9. Spencer H, Menczel J, Lewin I, Samachson J: "Absorption of Calcium in Osteoporosis," *Am J Med* 37:233, 1964

10. Sharp GS, Fister HW: "The Diagnosis and Treatment of Achlorhydria: Ten-Year Study." *J Am Geriatr Soc* 15:786, 1967

11. Oski FA: *Don't Drink Your Milk,* p. 60. Mollica Press, Syracuse, NY, 1983

4: Osteoporosis

1. Burckhardt P, Michel CH: "The Peak Bone Mass Concept." *Clin Rheumatology* 8:(Suppl. 2):16, 1989

2. Johnston CC, Longcope C: "Editorial: Premenopausal Bone Loss." *New Engl J Med* 323:1271, 1990

3. Lindsay R, et al: "Bone Response to Termination of Oestrogen Treatment." *Lancet* 1:1325, 1978

4. Nielsen, F: "Studies on the Relationship between Boron and Magnesium, Which Possibly Affects the Formation and Maintenance of Bones." *Magnesium Trace Elem* 9:61, 1990

5. Neilsen F, et al: "Effect of Dietary Boron on Mineral, Estrogen, and Testosterone Metabolism in Postmenopausal Women," *FASEB J* 1:394, 1987

6. National Research Council (U.S.): *Recommended Dietary Allowances.* 10th Ed. National Academy Press, Washington, D.C., 1989

7. Raloff J: "New Misgivings About Low Magnesium," *Science News* 133:356 June 4, 1988

8. Hyams DE, Ross EJ: "Scurvy, Megaloblastic Anaemia and Osteoporosis." *Br J Clin Pract* 17:332, 1963

9. Bland J: "Building Stronger Bones." *Delicious* July/August, 1988:12

10. Nielsen F, et al: "Effect of Dietary Boron on Mineral, Estrogen, and Testosterone Metabolism in Postmenopausal Women." *FASEB J* 1:394, 1987

11. Wenlock RW, Buss DH, Dixon EJ: "Trace Nutrients. 2. Manganese in British Food." *Brit J Nutr* 41:253, 1979

12. Robert D, et al: "Hypercalciuria During Experimental Vitamin K Deficiency in the Rat." *Calcif Tissue Int* 37:143, 1985

13. Bouckaert JS, Said AH: "Fracture Healing by Vitamin K." *Nature* 185:849, 1960

14. Gallagher JC, Riggs BL, DeLuca HF: "Effect of Treatment with Synthetic 1,25-dihydroxy-vitamin D in Postmenopausal Osteoporosis." *Clin Res* 27:366A, 1979

15. Holden JM, Wolf WR, Merta W: "Zinc and Copper in Self-Selected Diets." *J Am Diet Assoc* 75:23, 1979

16. Battstrom LE, Hultberg BL, Hardebo JE: "Folic Acid Responsive to Postmenopausal Homo-cysteinemia." *Metab* 34:1073, 1985

17. Recker RR: "Calcium Absorption and Achlor-hydria." *New Engl J Med* 313:(2):70, 1985

18. Nicar MJ, Pak CYC: "Calcium Bioavailability from Calcium Carbonate and Calcium Citrate." *J Clin Endoc Metab,* 61(2):391, 1985

5: Heart Disease

1. Coronary Drug Research Group: "Coronary Drug Project: Findings Leading to the Discontinuation of the 2.5mg/day Estrogen Group." *JAMA* 226:652, 1973

2. "Magnesium for Acute Myocardial Infarctions?" *Lancet* 338:667, 1991

3. Singh RB, et al: "Can Dietary Magnesium Modulate Blood Lipids." *J Amer Col Nutr* 9(5):527 (abst. 23), 1990

4. Taylor CB: "Spontaneously Occurring Angiotoxic

Derivatives of Cholesterol." *Amer J Clin Nutr* 32:40, 1979

5. Press R, et al: "The Effect of Chromium Picolinate on Serum Cholesterol and Apolipoprotein Fractions in Human Subjects." *West J Med* 152(1):41, 1990

6. Simonoff M: "Chromium Deficiency and Cardio-vascular Risk." *Cardiovasc Res* 18:591, 1984

7. Vinson J, et al: "Beneficial Effects of Antioxidant Vitamins on Lipids and Lipid Peroxidation." *J Amer Coll Nutr* 9(5):537 (abst. 55), 1990

6: Other Midlife Concerns: Breast Cancer, Diabetes, and Hypothyroidism

1. Steinberg KK, et al: "A Meta-Analysis of the Effect of Estrogen Replacement Therapy on the Risk of Breast Cancer." *JAMA* 265:1985, 1991

2. Seely S, Horrobin DF: "Diet and Breast Cancer: The Possible Connection with Sugar Consumption." *Med Hypoth* 11(3):319, 1983

Index

Recipe Index

About the Author

ANN LOUISE GITTLEMAN holds a master's degree in Nutritional Education from Columbia University. She has served as Chief Dietician of the Pediatric Clinic at NYU-Bellevue Medical Center; Nutritionist for the USDA's Women, Infants and Children Food Program at Yale University; and Nutrition Director at the Pritikin Longevity Center. She has been in private practice for over fifteen years and is currently a chairperson of the Department of Nutrition of the American Academy of Nutrition.

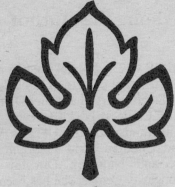